T0268329

BATTALION SURGEON

WILLIAM M. McCONAHEY, M.D.

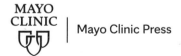

MAYO CLINIC | Mayo Clinic Press

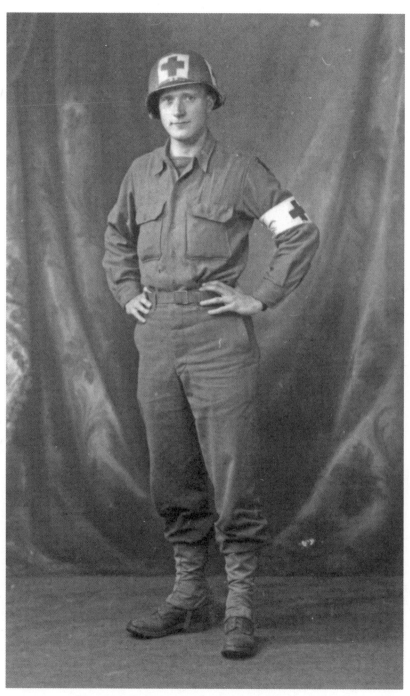

The author at Amneville, France, September 25, 1944.

MAYO CLINIC PRESS
200 First St. SW
Rochester, MN 55905
MCPress.MayoClinic.org

To stay informed about Mayo Clinic Press, please subscribe
to our free e-newsletter at **MCPress.MayoClinic.org**
or follow us on social media.

For bulk sales to employers, member groups and
health-related companies, contact
Mayo Clinic, 200 First St. SW, Rochester, MN 55905,
or send an email to SpecialSalesMayoBooks@mayo.edu.

Photographs provided by the family of
William M. McConahey, Jr., the U.S. Army Signal Corps and
MFMER. Cover photo courtesy of the U.S. Army Signal Corps.

ISBN: 979-8-887700-38-0

Library of Congress Control Number: 2023950533

Printed in the United States of America

**Proceeds from the sale of every book benefit medical research
and education at Mayo Clinic.**

For
ADRIENNE

This book is published with generous support from
John T. and Lillian G. Mathews,
Founding Benefactors of
Mayo Clinic Heritage Hall

FOREWORD

*V*ALUES, MORAL SCRUPLES, COMPASSION, UNWAVER-
ing devotion and the Greatest Generation.

These are the characteristics and descriptors of author
William M. McConahey, M.D., that stick with us after reading
his remarkable story. They also are attributes that those of us who
were privileged to serve as his colleagues at Mayo Clinic would
have used in describing Dr. McConahey, who made internation-
ally recognized contributions to advancing the care of patients
with thyroid and other endocrine disorders. He was a master cli-
nician at Mayo Clinic and one of the most honorable people we
would ever meet.

As his active duty was ending in 1945, he wrote this story of his
observations of his preceding two years in the U.S. Army as it
succeeded in the nearly impossible task of defeating Hitler's
powerful, entrenched army during World War II. His common-
man storytelling, written by an uncommonly great man, tells
the traumatic day-to-day stories of his 90th Division of General
George Patton's Third Army and its sweep across Europe. It is a
very personal story and describes the division's continuous battles
from the landing at Normandy's beaches two days after D-Day
through fighting in northern France, a diversion to Bastogne and
then across Germany to the Czech border. His perceptive observations bring the battles, victories and misery of it all to readers
with a palpable impact, as powerful and direct as the shock waves
from exploding German 88-mm shells as they fell into drenched
foxholes and sliced through the icebox forests of the Ardennes.

This book should be required reading for the various moral and
political factions that rend our national unity today. Dr. McConahey
was a man of honor in the most exceptional circumstances. He
provided care for everyone during the march across Europe,

regardless of their nationalities, morals or ethics. Moreover, he describes the extraordinary honor, fortitude and courage of his fellow soldiers, medics and physicians. They were devoted to their country and to those oppressed in Europe. Their virtues—and their travails and losses in battle—are set in granite. This book provides one of the very best descriptions of what it was like for these amazing men. We all should learn from them.

MARK A. WARNER, M.D.
EMERITUS EXECUTIVE DEAN,
MAYO CLINIC COLLEGE OF MEDICINE AND SCIENCE

Excerpts from the foreword to the original typewritten manuscript of this book, which Dr. McConahey wrote in the summer of 1945.

IN EXPLANATION

*T*HIS ACCOUNT OF MY EXPERIENCES AS A DOCTOR in combat in the Second World War is written for my family and any of my friends who may be interested.

Many sweeping concepts of the grand strategy of the conflict have been and will be written, but one who expects to find that here will be greatly disappointed. The war fought in division, corps, and army headquarters, where personal danger and discomfort were slight, was one of maps and lines and pins and shifting troops here and there—more like a fascinating game of chess. But the war I saw was one of mud and discomfort and suffering and death and terror and destruction.

I do not guarantee its accuracy. The overall picture is correct, but dates, places, and so forth may be wrong, since this was all written from memory. For security reasons, combat troops were ordered not to keep a journal during the war.

I make no claim to heroism because of this: I saw too many truly great heroes fight and die, ever to think that my efforts were heroic. The real heroes of this war were the infantry riflemen and the gallant company aid men.

This account, then, is a personal story of what I saw and did and thought from the day I began active duty with the army until the day I was separated from the Service.

WILLIAM M. McCONAHEY, M.D.

TABLE OF CONTENTS

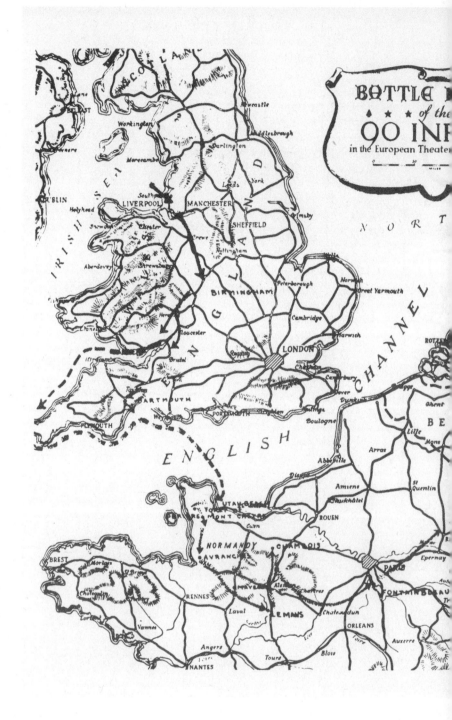

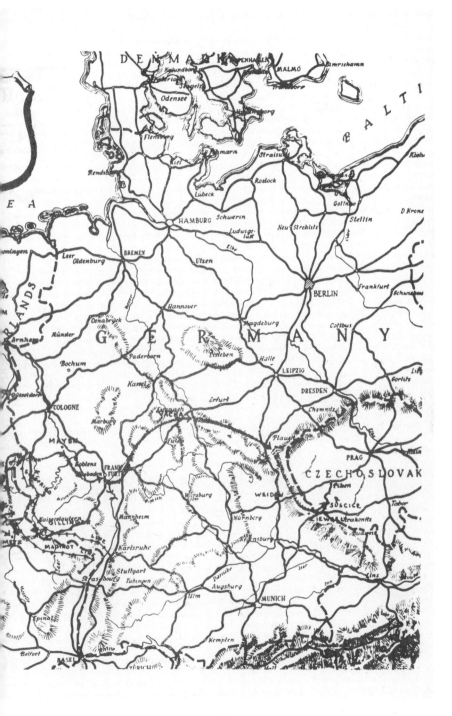

BATTALION SURGEON

PART ONE

Chapter One

INTRODUCTION TO THE ARMY

IT WAS ON JULY 17, 1943, THAT MY ARMY CAREER officially began, for on that day I entered active duty and began the six weeks' medical officers' training course at Carlisle Barracks, Pennsylvania. I was one of 500 doctors in the 33rd Officers' Training Battalion, and one of 1,500 at Carlisle, for every two weeks one group of 500 finished the six weeks' course and 500 more began. We were a green lot of medical officers, but before we left Carlisle we were well started on the way of all good medical officers. We had a full schedule of classes and drill periods from 8 a.m. to 5 p.m. six days a week, with frequent night classes and demonstrations. We had classes in military conduct and courtesies, logistics, military law, army organization, military strategy, sanitation, gas warfare, field medicine, map-reading and so forth. We had daily periods of close-order drill and calisthenics, a full-scale dress parade once a week, several distance marches, frequent gas-mask drills, and many demonstrations on how army medical installations function in the field. We went through the lethal gas chamber to be sure we could adjust our gas masks properly, ran the obstacle course, were "bombed" on cross-country hikes by cub planes' dropping small bags of flour, and watched a mock battle put on by the permanent troops stationed at the barracks. One night we had to follow a laid-out course by compass, observing complete blackout conditions. What a night that was! We stumbled in and out of ditches and felt our way through pitch-dark woods. On other nights we learned how to "freeze" when enemy aircraft drop flares, and how medical units work in blackout. There were also many fine training films shown to us on a great variety of subjects. The instruction at Carlisle and the many demonstrations were excellent—simply superb. I thought they did a fine job of getting all of us indoctrinated with the army and its ways.

My original orders were to report to Fort Bragg, North Carolina, upon completion of my course at Carlisle, for service with the 17th Airborne Division, which was supposed to be activated soon. However, this division never was activated, so I was ordered instead to Camp Carson, Colorado, to join the newly formed 71st Light Division.

A light division at that time was something new in the U.S. Army. It was patterned after the German light division, and was for fighting "in close and difficult terrain," to quote the War Department. The 71st Light Division was smaller than the standard triangular division. It had no heavy-weapons companies in its battalions; it had no cannon or antitank companies; the battalions were smaller; the headquarters groups were small; the artillery consisted solely of 75-mm. pack howitzers, and pack mules were the only means of transport besides some hand carts. In short, a light division was supposed to be a tough, well-knit group of hard-fighting men which could move and fight in the roughest, wildest kind of country. It was an experiment, and the 71st was one of two such light divisions started by the army to see if such outfits were practicable. The other one was the 89th Light Division (formed by revamping the old standard 89th). The 10th Mountain Division was also "light," but they were ski troops and were well established and no longer experimental.

I reported to Camp Carson on August 28, and began four and a half months of duty with the 71st Light Division. I was assigned to the 66th Infantry Regiment, and soon became the surgeon for the third battalion. It wasn't long before I learned that instead of being a group of tough fighting men, the division was filled with physical wrecks—castoffs from other units. Since this had been the last division activated in the whole U.S. Army, it had received many transfers from other outfits. Some of these transferred men were good, but too often they were the unwanted "eight-balls" and physical misfits of the transferring units. Sick call was "The Big Parade"; often we had 150 men a day on sick call from the 66th regiment. Not a few of these were "gold bricks" (malingerers), but many were truly physically disabled and unable to stand the stiff training program. "Trick" knees, bad ankles and feet, chronic low back strain, sore shoulders and so forth were common difficulties. We medical officers were in a tough position. In the first place, we had to weed out the malingerers from the others. Then we had to contend somehow with these chronically disabled. They weren't disabled enough for discharge; and they weren't acutely ill, so they couldn't be admitted to a hospital. Therefore, to the army, they were fit for full duty, and the company commanders were supposed to see that they did the job. Yet we medical officers knew that many of these fellows simply couldn't take it. We did the best we could; we put the worst cases in "quarters" when especially hard problems came along; we gave others "light duty" recommendations, and the "gold bricks" we sent back to full duty.

The training schedule was really a tough one. Long marches, many overnight problems and occasional three-day problems filled the full weeks. It was rugged work scrambling up and down the Rocky Mountains, carrying full packs. To carry the equipment for my battalion aid station I had two pack mules and two hand carts. We loaded the medical chests onto the mules, and the blanket set, splint set and litters onto the carts. These carts had to be pulled by hand, and how we sweated and griped as we pulled them over the steep, bumpy trails! But those mules! They were the worst of all. If they were the least bit overloaded they would refuse to budge until the extra few pounds were removed. Once, on a long march, they became frightened, and reared and bucked until the medical chests were thrown off and smashed, and the aid equipment was scattered over the countryside. On another occasion, during a regimental attack problem, I got the mules too far forward. They were silhouetted against the skyline in full view of the "enemy." A general saw them and came puffing up the hill, his face purple with rage.

"Who the hell has those God-damned mules?" he roared.

"I do, sir," I answered meekly.

"Well, get those jackasses the hell off this hilltop, and don't ever do that again!" he shrieked, waving his arms in the air and stamping the ground. After such a blasting it didn't take me long to drag my asses off that hilltop.

I wondered if we'd ease off a bit on the "rough stuff" when winter came, but no such luck. (I should have known the army better than that.) Instead of getting easier, the work got harder. They issued us fur jackets, arctic mittens, two pairs of wool trousers, arctic shoe pacs, eiderdown sleeping bags and special arctic tents; and the training program kept on, full steam ahead. Most of our days and many nights were spent in the field, in the snow and bitter cold of the Rockies. Many a time we'd leave camp about 3 a.m., march 10 miles or so before breakfast, so numb with cold we could hardly make it; and then after breakfast launch a full-scale, day-long "problem." At dark we'd throw our sleeping bags onto the snow and crawl in fully clothed for a chilly night. Sometimes we'd arise in the morning to find everything blanketed with several inches of new snow.

One night was so especially miserable that I never forgot it. We started out the day, as usual, with a cold, predawn march to the assembly point. Then our regiment "attacked" another "defending" regiment, and all day we "advanced." It warmed up during the day, so everyone took off his coat, and we piled the coats and sleeping bags up together and went on. About dark the "attack" stopped, and we were ordered to halt in place. Then the misery began. A subzero winter night descended on us, but we had no coats or sleeping bags. Because we were on a "problem" under "tactical conditions" we were not permitted to build fires or go back for our equipment. We were tired and we were stiff with cold; but all we could do was walk up and down, stamping our feet and swinging our arms to try to keep from freezing. That night we really "took apart" the army and some of its generals. Finally about midnight the colonel let us walk back, a few at a time, to get the equipment. I stumbled back the several miles in the darkness with some of my men to the place we had left the things, and we returned dragging as many coats and sleeping bags as we could carry. At last I got into my sleeping bag for a few cramped hours of rest before dawn, but I did not get warmed up all night. Although I spent many worse days and nights than that in combat, at this time these hardships in training seemed quite tough and unnecessary.

It puzzled us that we were being trained in cold weather for tropical fighting. It was no secret that the 71st was supposed to be a jungle division and was to see action against the Japs in the Pacific Theater. All the instruction classes we had were on Japanese tactics, jungle life, tropical medicine and so forth. We couldn't see the sense of training a jungle-bound outfit in the Rocky Mountains in winter, but we said, "That's the army."

Since we were heading toward the Pacific and the Japs, all medical personnel received rifle instruction. I spent quite a few hours on the firing range, and became a passable shot with the carbine and Garand rifle. I also went through the regimental close-combat course, which was a lot of fun. On the close-combat course one walked along a path and fired at dummies dressed like Japs which suddenly popped up in front of him or fell from trees at him. Another range I enjoyed was one at which men in foxholes scattered over a field raised man-sized targets on poles at random. The person on the firing line watched the field carefully and shot at every figure which bobbed up.

The infiltration course was one of those standard fixtures at most army camps. To go through this course a group of trainees gathered in a long trench on one side of a field, and at the blast of a whistle, crawled "over the top" and started to wriggle on their stomachs across the field through "shell holes" and under barbed wire, while dynamite charges exploded around them (to simulate bursting shells) and machine guns fired streams of bullets about 3 feet off the ground. All of us had to go through the course as a part of the "hardening for battle" process.

The battalions of the division were also taught how to attack pillboxes. Out some distance from camp had been built a group of pillboxes to represent a small part of the Siegfried Line, and these the men learned to assault. I saw our battalion going through the problem. I watched as the "attackers," under cover of a barrage of artillery, sneaked up to the fortifications, blew their way through the barbed wire with Bangalore torpedoes, and approached the concrete walls. Then, while bazooka men kept the gun ports "buttoned up," other members of the team advanced with dynamite charges and flame throwers, to finish off the objective. It was an interesting thing to watch, but I knew that in actual battle the casualties among these attackers would be enormous.

In the fall of 1943 I listened on the radio to President Roosevelt's speech in which he declared that the United States Army would invade the continent of Europe. How glad I was that I was with the 71st Division and would never have to assault that fearsome Atlantic Wall! But how little I realized! I never dreamed that I'd be in on that momentous task.

Shortly after I came to Camp Carson, my wife and five-month-old son came out to join me. For a while we lived in tourist cabins, but before long we were able to rent a house in partnership with a fellow regimental officer—a chaplain—and his wife and two-year-old daughter. Our "house partners" were Finley W. Tinnin, his wife, Eloise, and little Linda, from Louisiana. The house was an old lodge in a beautiful location part way up Cheyenne Mountain, above the Broadmoor Hotel. From our lodge we looked down on Colorado Springs, the Broadmoor and out across miles of plains to the east. It was a beautiful view. We thoroughly enjoyed our stay in Colorado. We loved Colorado Springs, the fine climate and the beautiful Rocky Mountains. In company with the Tinnins we saw many of the scenic points of that area—the Garden of the Gods, the Royal Gorge, the Skyline Drive, Cripple Creek, the Manitou Incline, Pike's Peak (via the cog railway) and many others. We also spent some time in Denver, and once I even climbed Pike's Peak with three other officers. It was an interesting experience, living in Colorado, and we enjoyed it greatly.

I had a 10-day leave the first part of January, 1944, which we spent right around Colorado Springs. When I returned to camp at the end of my vacation, I found things at a fever pitch. The division had just been alerted for a move the end of the month to California for extensive maneuvers on the Hunter Liggett reservation. From then on, things were in an uproar, as we prepared for

8

the move. At home, too, things were in confusion, as we tried to plan for Adrienne and Billy to move to California. Since I'd have to accompany the men on the troop train, Adrienne would have to drive across the Rockies to California alone, with a nine-month-old baby. And once she got there, where could she go? Housing around all army centers was at a premium, we well knew. We worried and planned long hours about what to do.

However, our turmoil was all in vain, for about a week before we were scheduled to leave for California, I suddenly got orders to join the 90th Infantry Division waiting at Fort Dix, New Jersey, to go overseas. So, after three days of intensive packing and checking out at various places in Camp Carson, I was ready to leave, and we started east through a heavy snow which had fallen the night before. Since I did not have to report at Fort Dix until February 4, we were able to stop off in Coshocton, Ohio, for a few days' visit with Adrienne's family. I was glad of this, but wondered if I'd ever see them again.

Chapter Two

ATLANTIC CROSSING

O<small>N FEBRUARY 3, I LEFT COSHOCTON FOR FORT DIX,</small> accompanied by my wife. Billy's grandparents kindly offered to keep him for a while, so we left him in Coshocton. We went by train to Philadelphia, spent the night there, and the next day took a bus toward Fort Dix. Since we knew how impossible it usually was to find a room on short notice near an army camp, we got off the bus at Mt. Holly, a little town 10 miles or so from the camp, and secured a room in a small, dingy, rundown hotel. I kissed Adrienne goodbye and started on for camp, not knowing whether I'd ever see her again or not. I had no idea whether the 90th Division was still preparing for shipment or whether it was already all set to sail. Much to my relief, when I signed in at headquarters, I learned that we'd be in the States a while longer. I was assigned to the 357th Infantry Regiment, and then was told that since this was Saturday evening, I could leave now and report back for duty Monday morning. Happily I returned to Mt. Holly for a nice week end with Adrienne.

On Monday I began my work with the 90th. The officers of the medical detachment were nine. Four of these had been with the division a long time: Major Marion Brown (detachment commander), Captain "Tony" Dominski, Captain "Vic" Di Leo and Captain Lloyd Blackwell (one of the regimental dentists). The other five had just been transferred in from other divisions: Captain Ed Rapp (the other dentist), Lieut. (later Captain) Jack Gable, Captain

John Boccaccio, Captain Ted Bruce and I. We got along well together throughout the war. I was originally assigned to the third battalion to work with Tony Dominski, but shortly after D-Day I became surgeon of the second battalion.

My duties at this time involved helping with sick call, conducting close-order drill and calisthenics for the men, taking the detachment on long marches, inspecting the men's equipment, supervising the packing of the medical supplies and the personal goods of the men and so on. One day I was asked to demonstrate some white phosphorus grenades for the men, so I took three grenades and marched the detachment a couple of miles from camp. I got the men behind me, pulled the pin from one grenade and flung it as far as I could. With a roar it exploded, throwing out great streamers of flaming white phosphorus, and in a few seconds the field was ablaze in a hundred or so places. For a moment or so we stood transfixed, and then, "coming to," we all rushed in and stamped out the fires. Then I wondered what to do with the other two grenades remaining. I didn't want to carry them back, and besides, I didn't know where to turn them in. Finally, I decided to explode them, too. This I did, and after each one we stamped out fires. I was afraid of starting extensive grass fires, and for a few minutes it looked as though that would happen, but it did not.

As it turned out, we left Fort Dix the middle of March, but of course, none of us knew that in advance. We had to be ready to pull out anytime. Adrienne stayed in Mt. Holly a couple of weeks, and then returned to Coshocton, but I saw her on the next four week ends. Once she came to Philadelphia, twice we met in Pittsburgh, and once I went to Cleveland. Each time I'd leave her to return to camp, I wouldn't know whether I'd see her the next week end or whether we'd ship out before then.

Finally, of course, came the last goodbye, but we didn't know it. We had had a wonderful week end in Philadelphia together. When I put her on the train in North Philadelphia Sunday evening, March 12, to go back to Ohio we said the usual thing, "Well, maybe this is goodbye, but then maybe we'll meet again next week end." I watched the train leave, and then dejectedly walked back to the bus station for a bus back to Fort Dix. When I got back to camp, there was the expected order: "The 90th Division is sealed into camp as of midnight tonight. No personnel will be permitted to leave camp for any purpose." Well, that was that. At last we were going overseas, but none of us knew yet to what embarkation point we'd proceed.

Monday morning further orders were issued. The division would begin entraining on Wednesday, March 15. The 357th Infantry would leave on Thursday. Since I was named surgeon for one of the troop trains, I did not travel with the medical detachment, but went on the train carrying the second battalion. We loaded onto the cars, but had only a short ride, for we went to Camp Kilmer, New Jersey, not far away. Camp Kilmer was one of the largest embarkation points on the east coast. After we arrived there, I rejoined the medical detachment.

Then began a strange but very interesting six days. How they ever processed us in so short a time I'll never know, but my hat's off to the Army Transportation Corps for the magnificent job they did. The whole thing moved easily and progressively, like well-oiled machinery. With thousands upon thousands of troops flowing through the camp on their way overseas every week, the task of the Transportation Corps was tremendous. We attended lectures and demonstrations on how to live at sea in a lifeboat or on a life raft, we saw moving pictures on how to abandon ship if we went down at sea, we practiced climbing down a rope cargo net into a lifeboat, we were issued the new-type gas mask and learned how to use it, and we officers inspected very thoroughly the equipment of every man in the detachment. Then we also had to give the first of a series of three typhus shots to every man in the regiment, as well as a quick general physical examination.

Finally, all these preparations were completed, and we got our orders to proceed to the harbor on March 22. The division was to be carried on 21 trains, leaving every 20 minutes, starting about noon. I was named car commander of one of the railroad cars carrying the medical detachment. In order to assure quick loading of the train we carefully practiced the standard loading procedure, until all the men understood it. Then we wrote numbers in chalk on each man's helmet corresponding with seat numbers in the cars so we could keep track of everyone easier and also tell at a glance if things were in order. When our turn came, we piled our duffle bags on trucks, marched to the camp railyards, got our baggage off the trucks there and climbed into the train.

It was dusk as the train pulled out for a slow, 2-hour trip to Jersey City. No words could express adequately our mixed emotions as we sat in that car. Some of the fellows tried to laugh and sing and joke in a nervous sort of way, but most of us simply sat silently staring out into the darkness and thinking. It was too late to turn back now. What lay ahead? What would the sea trip across be like? Where were we going? What would it feel like to be in battle? How many of us would never return, and how many would come back maimed?

Crack passenger trains sped by, with the lighted diners and club cars filled with gay, chatting civilians. What did they know of war? Shortages, rationing and newspaper headlines. Were they perhaps headed for Chicago for a big week end while we were bound for the cold Atlantic? Oh well; so what?

The train stopped near the waterfront in Jersey City, and we quickly piled off. Struggling along with our heavy duffle bags and other equipment we walked as fast as we could to a large automobile ferry. When it was filled with troops, it started off across the harbor. After a trip of half an hour or so, it pulled up to a dock and, looming up above us, we saw a large passenger ship which we knew must be our transport. We marched off the ferry into the huge shed on the pier. The whole scene seemed strange and unreal and like a dream. While bright lights blazed down from the roof and an army swing band blared forth the *Twelfth Street Rag,* we checked off our names on a list held by a clerk and walked up the long gangplank and onto the ship.

Once on board ship, I located my quarters and found that I was sharing a cabin with Captain Mangnuson. Then I went to an officers' meeting. Here we were told that we were on the *Dominion Monarch*, a fine new British luxury liner. She had been built just before the war for the England-to-New Zealand run, and had made only one trip before war broke out. Since then she had been transporting men and supplies all over the world. She was one of five ships, from a convoy of 15, which had survived concerted air and submarine attacks to get through to Malta to break the siege in the summer of 1943, I believe. We were not told where we were going, but strong hints were dropped that it would be England. There were about 3,000 men on board, we were informed, with the majority being our 357th regiment.

A little later I went to see if I could help the enlisted men of the medical detachment get settled, but they were all set. All cabins and salons had been removed from the lower decks, and here the enlisted men were quartered together. It was quite a trick to get so many men onto a ship, but a good job of it had been done. The boys slept in hammocks which they put up at night and took down in the morning. After talking with our boys for a few minutes, I went back and went to bed.

When I awoke in the morning, the ship was under way, sailing out of New York harbor. I dressed and went outside on deck in the morning mist to see the Statue of Liberty and to watch the skyline of New York disappear astern. When we got outside the harbor we picked up the rest of the convoy and started east. What a sight it was to see our huge convoy spread out almost as far as the horizon! There were about 60 vessels in all, according to my count. The convoy leader was the light cruiser, *U.S.S. Cincinnati;* there were nine or ten troop transports (including the Canadian Pacific Railroad's *Duchess of Bedford* and two of the *Castle* liners); there was an aircraft carrier delivering a load of partly assembled planes to England; there was an oil tanker for the refueling of the submarine chasers; there was a host of merchantmen; and of course there were many destroyers and submarine chasers dodging in and out.

We sailed from New York on March 23 and landed in Liverpool on April 4, a trip of 12 days by way of a weaving, circuitous route. For the first few days out of New York we were escorted by a blimp and flights of land-based planes, and when we neared England, British planes circled overhead. As far as I know, the trip across was uneventful except that we had a rather bad storm. It was really an unusually heavy blow, and our ship rolled and pitched violently. Great numbers of the boys became seasick, but as usual, my stomach behaved. It was a boring trip, however, for I had little to do. I helped some in the ship's infirmary, read mystery stories and walked the decks. Of course, all of us wore our life preservers all our waking hours, and laid them carefully beside us at night. Abandon-ship drill and anti-aircraft practice broke the monotony a bit each day. And all over the ship money changed hands rapidly. In the officers' lounge poker games involving hundreds of dollars went on day and night, while in the enlisted men's quarters crap games were played constantly, with sometimes several thousand dollars depending on one roll of the dice.

At last our voyage came to an end. On April 4 we sighted the British Isles, and glad we were to see the shore! The convoy broke up and we headed for Liverpool, where we were to disembark. Late that afternoon our ship slipped into her berth, while a British band standing on the wharf welcomed us to England by playing *The Stars and Stripes Forever*.

Chapter Three

ENGLAND

*J*ENJOYED MY BRIEF STAY IN ENGLAND, IN SPITE OF the black prospect of D-Day in the background. I liked the English countryside and I found the British people quite pleasant and friendly. They had suffered greatly from the war already, yet none of them complained. They were all pulling together for our common victory.

I left the ship, along with part of the medical detachment, before dawn on the morning of April 5, and walked to the a near-by railway shed. There we loaded into railway cars for a trip southeastward. This was my first encounter with European railway trains, and how strange they looked to me! They seemed so small and almost toylike when compared to American trains. Then, too, the division of the passenger cars into compartments was a new thing to me.

When we were all on, the train started off across England. Soon the sun came up, and what pretty sights greeted our eyes! Well-ordered fields, shimmering in the morning mist, and towns and villages, with smoke curling from many tiled chimneys, slid past the windows of our train as it puffed along. We learned that we were headed for a camp near Birmingham in the Midlands (the industrial center of England).

About 1000 hours the train stopped and we got off. A convoy of army trucks was waiting to drive us to the camp which was to be our home for the next 6 or 7 weeks. How strange it was to be driving on the left side of the road, but then this was England. The camp to which we went was located on a part of the grounds of Kinlet Hall, a huge private estate. It had just been laid out, and there were few buildings on it. We lived in tents, and the occasional Quonset huts here and there were used for aid stations, mess halls, kitchens and C.P.'s.* My "home" was a two-man tent, which I shared with Tony Dominski. As usual, the English spring was cold and rainy, so we were none too comfortable; and of course the camp was a sea of mud most of the time.

I was appointed camp sanitary officer soon after we arrived. Most of the camp was in good order, but one thing bothered me considerably—the latrines. Instead of having deep-pit latrines, well protected from flies, as was our custom in the U.S. Army, the British apparently preferred the miserable "honey-bucket" system. Under each seat was a bucket, which was emptied every day or so by a local farmer, and hauled away for fertilizer. Some spilling on the ground was inevitable; some of the buckets overflowed; often a stream of urine ran from each latrine; swarms of flies appeared; and after his collections, the farmer drove his truck across camp with feces-mixed urine dribbling from the back. It was an inexcusably insanitary arrangement, but in spite of my vigorous protests, I was unable to have those latrines abandoned and deep-pit ones dug. I was informed that there was some ruling preventing the digging of holes in the ground here, but this was a flimsy excuse. This part of our sanitation was disgraceful.

As soon as we got settled in camp, we were informed that we were about to embark on an extensive training program, and that none of us could be farther than a 3-hour journey from camp at any time. At Kinlet Hall were regimental headquarters and the 2nd and 3rd battalions of the 357th Infantry. And train we did! From reveille at 0600 to retreat at 1700 hours (5:00 p.m.) we worked hard. We had calisthenics, gas-mask drill, litter drill and so forth; and every other afternoon a grueling hike. At first the marches were simply long conditioning hikes (15 miles) at a normal speed, but then we started "speed" hikes, on which we were supposed to

---

* Command posts.

go 5 miles in 1 hour and 9 miles in 2 hours. These speed hikes are fiendish inventions, for at 5 miles an hour the cadence is faster than a walk and slower than a dog trot. On these marches (with full packs, of course) the battalion would be strung out for miles, as man after man fell out and straggled along behind as best he could. These were killing on me. "Shin splints" developed on the first one, and from then on every step I took at this fast pace was agony. I dreaded these affairs, yet I went on every one. Had I not been an officer, I'm sure I would have dropped out, but I couldn't let my men down that way. So I struggled through them, biting the chin strap of my helmet and sweating profusely. I never lagged or fell out, but at the end of each one my anterior tibial muscles were paralyzed so that I was unable to dorsiflex (raise) my feet, and I'd end the march slapping my feet down on the road like a tabetic person. About this time I began hoping for D-Day to come!

In spite of our active training schedule, I was able to see a little of this part of England, for we had evenings and Sundays off. The nearest village was Bewdley, a quaint little town with not much in it in the way of entertainment. The nearest town of any size was Kidderminster, about 14 miles away, and the large city of Birmingham was about 25 miles away. Trucks from camp went to these places every evening and on Sunday, so frequently I spent evenings in Kidderminster or Birmingham. During the war, England was on double-summer time, so it was 10:30 or 11:00 p.m. before it got dark. The blackouts were strange to us at first, but we soon got used to pitch-dark streets and dim slits of light on vehicles for headlights. It was strange to walk the streets of a great city after dark and hear the hubbub of many people going by, and yet see almost no one. One Sunday I went to Coventry and on another Sunday I spent a fascinating afternoon at Stratford-on-Avon.

I had become acquainted with a few English families and found them to be delightful people. Although they were more reserved than the exuberant Americans, they were warm friends and seemed to be genuinely interested in us. I admired their uncomplaining attitude. Not only had they gone through the blitz, but also they had done without so many things for years. "Shortages" were legion. There were few automobiles, very little gasoline for business travel and no gasoline at all for pleasure driving. The people got one egg a month, but never any oranges. Clothing was scarce, and soap and tobacco were luxury items. We American soldiers in England fared better than the civilians, although we were strictly rationed on candy, soap, tobacco, razor blades and chewing gum. The English children never before had had chewing gum, so they besieged us all with, "Any gum, chum?"

One of my less enjoyable tasks during the war was censoring the mail of my men. The letters of all enlisted men written in a combat zone had to be read by an officer before they were mailed, so that no information of value to the enemy would slip through. From the time we left Fort Dix until the end of the war I read the letters written by the men in my medical section, and what a boring job that was! Before I had been at it long, however, I learned to skim a paragraph at a glance, and without reading it fully, to tell whether it contained any "restricted" material. I was happy indeed when mail censorship was ended in Europe after V-E Day.

For some reason, I had never thought that I would be in on D-Day. I knew the 90th Division had had no amphibious training, so I thought we'd perhaps sit in England for a month or two after D-Day and then go in after the worst fighting was over. How wrong I was! One evening late in April, our battalion commander called the officers together for one of our frequent officers' meetings, but this was no routine gathering.

"Men," he said, "I have just come from a meeting with the corps commander. He tells us that we are 'on the first team.' That's all I can say, but you know what that means."

Yes, we knew—D-Day! My heart sank into my boots when I heard those words. It looked as though we were in for a rough time.

Frequently we listened to the radio in the evenings. It seemed strange to twist the dial and hear so many stations "jammed" off the air. I had never heard any radio jamming in the States, of course. The Germans used a peculiar musical jamming. On the same wave length as that of certain enemy stations they did not want to be heard, they would broadcast monotonous series of musical notes over and over, thus effectively drowning out the unwanted radio stations.

We often tuned in on "Axis Sally" and her regular evening broadcast. She played many excellent recordings of popular American songs, which included a lot of Bing Crosby's. In between songs she'd shoot us the propaganda like this: "Hello, all you Yanks over there. How are you tonight? Homesick? Of course you are, and no wonder, now that you are here to fight England's war for her and to die for John Bull. Don't worry, Yanks, Britain will not allow any Englishman to die on the Atlantic Wall. That's for you! Why are you over here, Yanks? You know why—to make more money for the Jewish capitalists and Bolshevik warmongers in America, with *your* blood. But let's not talk about such unpleasant things. Now we'll play an old favorite for you, *Two Cigarettes in the Dark*. Remember it? And remember those warm summer nights when you sat close to her and she whispered, 'I love you' and nestled closer in your arms? Now she's over there and you are here, and you'll never see her again, for you are going to die. You will die, you know, on our impregnable Atlantic Wall. Now here's the music."

After Axis Sally's program would come a violent speech by some leather-lunged male, which would be something like this: "So you Yanks are sweating out D-Day! You wonder when it will come, don't you? Well, we don't care when it comes; we are ready for you. We are waiting to hurl your corpses back into the sea. You can never break through our Atlantic Wall. It is impregnable everywhere. We are ready and waiting. We have a date with you on D-Day. And what does D stand for? *(Voice rising to a screaming crescendo.)* D for Death on the beaches of Dieppe and Dunkirk!"

"Lord Haw-Haw," the renegade Englishman who broadcast propaganda for the enemy, could be heard on the radio every evening. His "Views of the News" was mostly concerned with strikes and draft-dodgers in America, entirely fictitious accounts of glorious German victories in Russia and Italy, stories about "rich Jewish capitalists" and "Russian Bolsheviks," scandalous gossip about Allied leaders, the futility and hopelessness of the Allied efforts, the uselessness of the "death of so many Yanks for England's greed," and so forth.

During my stay in England the *Luftwaffe* never paid a visit any-where close to us, but occasionally did bomb cities some distance away. One night in May I awoke to hear the distant rumble of fall-ing bombs and the crash of anti-aircraft fire. I knew that the enemy planes would not come our way that night, but for a long time I lay awake, staring into the darkness and thinking. I won-dered what it would be like to be in battle, and especially how I'd react. Would I measure up to the test or would I be less than a man? One of these days I'd know.

We had two great speculative pastimes, one of which might be called "Who else is here?" We didn't like the idea of being too much alone in this big show, and we longed for plenty of company. We hoped there were dozens of American divisions over here. Time and again we'd name over the divisions we knew were in England. We'd say, "Well, the 1st, 2nd, 4th, 9th, 29th, 30th and 90th infan-try divisions are here, and the 5th, 6th and 7th Armored, and—" It helped us to think that "our team" was a big one.

The other great speculation was *"When* will it be D-Day, and *where* will it be?" We could see events moving swiftly and inexo-rably toward the great climax, but how soon it would be we could only guess. Not until a few days before June 6 did we know that D-Day was at last at hand. As the days and weeks went by the ten-sion built up until it was tremendous, and one felt as though he'd explode from the inward pressure. We also wondered where we'd land on the continent. Most of us thought it would probably be somewhere on the French coast, but we wondered about Norway and the Balkans.

One comforting factor was the Allied air power. I never saw a Jerry plane over England (although every night a few would sneak over to bomb here and there), but at almost any time during the day one could look skyward and see one or more Allied planes in the air. At night the roar of their motors was nearly continuous. American Liberators and Fortresses and British Lancasters and Wellingtons were constantly going and coming on bombing mis-sions, while Spitfires, Thunderbolts, Mustangs and Lightnings flew fighter cover. It was truly awe-inspiring.

The 90th Division was a part of the Third Army from the first, but for the Normandy campaign we were attached to the First Army (since the Third Army didn't take the field until after Normandy). Shortly before D-Day we heard three of our leaders speak, on three different occasions. Major General Lawton Collins, the commander of the corps to which we were attached, addressed us at Kinlet Hall. Then later the officers of the division traveled to Birmingham to hear General (then Lieutenant General) Omar Bradley. He impressed us very greatly with his sincerity, quiet confidence and genuine friendliness. He gave us a fatherly sort of talk and looked more like a midwest banker than the great military genius he is. We loved Bradley and felt we could trust him all the way.

And finally, General (then Lieutenant General) George S. Patton addressed us, and that was quite an occasion. All the commissioned and noncommissioned officers of the division were assembled to hear him. As his shiny limousine drove up we were called to attention. The car stopped and out stepped Patton. He handed his natty-looking, long gray overcoat to an aide and then mounted the platform. The tall general looked quite impressive in his polished boots, breeches, snappy jacket with banks of colorful ribbons and lacquered helmet-liner with the three gleaming stars of a lieutenant general riveted to the front. Then followed the most fiery, "fightingest" harangue I have ever heard. It was a harangue, all right, but it was masterful. The language was far from parlor English, for he cursed and swore at a great rate, but he really put the speech across. Patton was an expert at inciting men to a high fighting pitch. A few of his phrases which I recall were as follows.

"When the Krauts drop artillery shells on you, don't stop; keep moving forward! The bastards always lengthen their range and never shorten it."

"You've heard it said, 'Dig foxholes or die.' That's bullshit! Don't dig 'em too deep or you can't get out of 'em, and they'll turn into your grave!"

"We're going to kick the sons of bitches up one hill and down another, clear to Berlin!"

23

"Don't worry about being killed. You all won't die, and the medics do wonders for the wounded."

"When your kids ask, 'What did you do in the war?' you can say proudly, 'I was there!' instead of having to say, 'All I did was shovel shit in Illinois.'"

"There are yellow-bellied sons of bitches in every outfit. When you find them, don't let them run away. Make the bastards do their share of the fighting or stick a bayonet into their guts!"

"You probably wonder how to identify Kraut and Allied planes. Don't bother with that. If a plane shoots at you, shoot back."

"Let's hurry up and beat the Boche before those bastards in the Pacific finish off the Japs. We want to get over there, too; it's a duty to fight the Germans, but it's a pleasure to fight the Japs!"

"Old Blood and Guts" really lived the part.

We were given as detailed training as possible. We had demonstrations of German uniforms and weapons. We were also told what to do if we were captured—how much to say, how to conduct ourselves, what tricks the enemy might pull and how to escape. We were carefully drilled on how to distinguish American from German paratroopers, and were briefed on how air-borne troops operate.

Sick call became somewhat of a problem as the time wore on. We wanted to be sure that we did not take any physically unfit men along on the invasion, yet we didn't want to let the "gold bricks" wriggle out of it. So it was quite a responsibility for us battalion surgeons to keep a sharp eye on the health of the men in the battalion.

One certain warm, quiet evening in May has remained in my memory, and sometimes this memory returns to haunt me. All the officers of the regiment had been assembled for a weekly meeting, as was the custom. On this evening our beloved and respected regimental commanding officer, Colonel Sheehy, addressed us. The silver-haired colonel, who soon was to lead us into battle, arose and said in a quiet, dignified voice, "Gentlemen, we have heard these last few days what to do if we are captured. It even sounds like fun to be captured and to escape, but that's not the case. Let us resolve not to become prisoners. We are here to fight and win a war, not to give up to the enemy. Let us be known as a fighting regiment, rather than as surrendering cowards. Fight always, then, and don't surrender. It isn't so bad to die."

Within 24 hours of his first action the gallant colonel was dead, cut down by Kraut machine gunners while he was at the front of his men; and before the Normandy campaign was over, the majority of the officers who heard his words that spring evening were dead or badly wounded.

The second week of May we got orders to move, but we didn't know where. We did know, however, that the "big day" was fast approaching, for we were ordered to take only what we could carry on our backs and to pack all other belongings in our foot lockers for storage in Liverpool for "the duration." On May 13 we moved about 100 miles southwest to the quaint little Welsh village of Chepstow, not far from the city of Bristol and the sea. We were quartered in a camp built on and around a race track just outside the village. There were many interesting sights to see around here on our Sundays and evenings off—the ancient wall around Chepstow, a medieval castle (which Oliver Cromwell besieged but could not capture), the ruins of Tintern Abbey, the beautiful Wye River, parts of the old Roman wall and the interesting cities of Bristol, Cardiff and Newburyport. My quarters while we were here were in a room underneath one of the grandstands at the race track. Our training program these days was light, and consisted mainly of marches and packing.

One night Jerry planes bombed Bristol, passing directly over our camp on their bombing runs. Our men were forbidden to fire, for to do so might reveal the camp to the enemy.

Sunday, May 28, I was away from camp most of the day, as I usually was on my day off. When I returned about dusk, I learned that the camp was now sealed, and none of us could leave it again for any purpose. The next day the officers of the regimental and battalion staffs were taken to a secret room and carefully briefed on the D-Day plans. They were shown on a relief map made of sand where we would land, and they were told exactly what we were supposed to do. Since I was not included in this group of briefed officers, and since they were sworn to secrecy, I still did not know where we'd invade the coast.

During the next several days we were busy waterproofing equipment for the landing operations. Since a gas attack by the enemy against our beachhead was feared, we carried gas masks, and these had to be carefully waterproofed and yet kept handy for quick "dewaterproofing" if the need should arise. We were also issued chemically treated, gas-resistant fatigue suits to be worn over our woolen uniforms on D-Day. For aid equipment on the beach we were given large, cylindrical, waterproofed, heavy cardboard cases in which 155-mm. artillery shells had been packed. Now the cases contained plasma, morphine, bandages and so forth. All vehicles were also completely waterproofed so that they could be driven into and even under water. A gum substance was packed over all parts which water would harm, and a long tube was run up about 6 feet above the motor from the air intake of the carburetor. Now the vehicles would not need a dock for unloading, but could be driven off the landing barges, into the water and onto the shore. This was a great surprise to Jerry.

On one afternoon during this week the regiment took a practice march with full equipment to see how we'd fare on a "dress rehearsal." We wore our wool O.D. uniforms and over them the airtight, gas-resistant fatigue suits, and we carried full packs and all our aid-station equipment (litters, blanket sets, water, splint sets and so forth). The battalion companies carried all their equipment, too—machine guns, rifles, mortars, B.A.R.'s, full ammunition and so forth. It was a blistering hot day, and the march was grueling. We suffered acutely from the heat and especially from the airtight, gasproof fatigues. Not only would they keep gas out, but they also kept air out and heat and perspiration in. A few men fell out during the march, but the big trouble came just after we got back to camp. Hardly had we returned when men began dropping down all over the place with heat exhaustion and severe heat cramps. We physicians and our aid men were nearly exhausted ourselves, but we had a lot of work to do to take care of the ill soldiers. It worried me considerably that we had fared so badly on the dress rehearsal. I feared that these uniforms would give us much trouble in combat. However, my fears were not realized, for

26

June in France was cold and wet, and the fatigue suits gave us some protection against both the cold and the water.

On Friday, June 2, our jeep drivers were ordered to leave with the jeeps to load the vehicles onto landing barges. Then we knew that D-Day was nearly at hand. We were first ordered to be ready to leave camp on Saturday, but the time was changed to early Sunday morning. This probably was caused by the delaying of the invasion date by one day. Most of us still knew nothing about the part we were to play in the invasion or when it would be. Now that events were obviously approaching a climax, the tension built up to almost unbearable heights. Nerves were taut, but tempers did not flare. Instead, a powerful bond of comradeship and helpfulness in the face of impending danger was born.

For the last two nights in camp, Friday and Saturday, Tony and I moved over from the officers' section to live with the men of our medical battalion. We wanted to be close to them and give them all the moral support we could.

Friday and Saturday I got all of my equipment in order, took the last shower I'd have for many weeks, and washed a few clothes. Saturday evening I wrote my "last letter" to Adrienne. There were so many things I wanted to say, but how could I put them in a letter? I wanted to write the proper letter in case I did not live to write another, but I couldn't put my thoughts in words. So I wrote a note and then went to bed, wondering how I'd react in battle and whether I'd be a credit to myself and my country.

PART TWO

Chapter Four

INTO FRANCE

*A*BOUT SUNRISE SUNDAY, JUNE 4, WE AROSE, dressed, ate breakfast and formed into ranks with full equipment. Then we marched out of camp to the troop trains several miles away. A few raindrops splattered down from leaden skies on the long columns of silent soldiers marching thoughtfully through the streets of Chepstow. A few early risers glanced at the heavily laden troops, but paid little heed to them. The people of Chepstow had long ago become accustomed to the coming and going of American troops at all hours of the day and night. But we knew. This was the real thing. Our days of training and practicing were over. Soon the "big show" would begin, and we of the 90th Infantry Division were on the first team. Although the morning was cool, I was sweating, and no wonder. I wore a wool undershirt, a wool O.D. uniform, a gas-resistant fatigue suit and a field jacket; and I carried a fully packed musette bag, entrenching shovel, full canteen, gas mask, first-aid kit, shelter-half and a waterproofed paper 155-mm. shell case filled with medical supplies.

Soon we reached the train, quickly loaded into the coaches and started the short journey to Bristol. There I got the medical section off the train, lined up and marched onto our invasion ship, the army transport *S. S. Bienville.* Tony Dominski was busy elsewhere, so I got the men settled in their crowded quarters in one of the holds. Then I went to find my quarters. Tony and I were sharing a six-man room with four other captains: Captain Allen Calhoun

(French interpreter and CIC*), Captain Grant (division staff), a chemical warfare officer, and one other. The food was excellent on the ship, and we took it easy, eating, sleeping and reading. On Monday (the next day) the *Bienville* put out to sea to the rendezvous area off Swansea. There we got a look at our invasion armada, and what a sight! hundreds of ships—troop transports, freighters, tankers, destroyers, minesweepers, Liberty ships. Many of the freighters towed captive balloons (barrage balloons) high above them to keep strafing and bombing planes high.

On Monday we were given a thorough briefing. D-Day probably would be Tuesday; we would land on D plus 2; the place of landing was the Cotentin (Cherbourg) Peninsula; the objective was Cherbourg; the 4th Division was going in first; and the paratroopers would land behind the beaches. Well, at at last we knew, but the knowledge gave me a funny feeling in my stomach. D plus 2! My gosh, that was darn soon. As an assistant battalion surgeon with the infantry, I had no illusions about the danger and difficulty of my job. We pored over maps and air photographs of the areas we were going to attack, getting all details worked out. Those of us who were in positions in which we might be captured were issued aids in escaping. We were given a map of western Europe printed on a piece of silk about the size of a pocket handkerchief, a tiny steel file about an inch long, and a little half-inch-long piece of magnetized steel which always pointed north when balanced on the point of a pin (to be used as a compass).

Tuesday morning we awoke to the news that "the show" was on. All day we listened eagerly to reports coming in over the radio. Late in the day our huge convoy weighed anchor and started for France, closely hugging the southern coast of England. That evening we listened to the King of England give his inspiring D-Day address. The ship's wireless picked it up, and it was put on the public-address system. Wednesday was a nerve-racking day. We knew we'd be landing the next day, and you could almost see men tightening up nervously. Large crowds attended the religious services held by the chaplains each night on the ship, and

* Counter Intelligence Corps.

everyone did a great deal of quiet thinking and praying. About dark the submarine alerts began, and all night long we heard and felt the dull, booming thuds of the depth charges dropped by the destroyer escorts.

Thursday morning dawned bright and clear, and soon after sunup we sighted the Normandy shore and the awe-inspiring invasion fleet along the coast. As we drew closer and took our appointed places, the whole scene unfolded. Mighty American and British battleships and heavy cruisers lay offshore, hurling broadside after broadside at Nazi-held forts still resisting, and at targets farther inland. Here and there white geysers of water leaped up where shells from shore batteries splashed around the Allied ships. Now and then a vessel would hit a mine and sink, while surrounding boats took off the personnel. There were hundreds and hundreds of ships of all sizes dotting the sea, and in and out dashed the LST's, LCP's, ducks and so forth, unloading men and equipment from the big ships. Now and then boats loaded with wounded men passed us on the way from the shore to hospital ships—a grim reminder to us all. In the sky droned squadron after squadron of Allied planes flying cover for us. About noon it became our turn to unload. We adjusted our special carbon-dioxide life belts, put our equipment on in such a manner that it could be shed quickly if we fell into the water, and clambered over the side and down the cargo net into the LCP tossing on the waves below. I was leading the medical section again, since Tony was in a different boat, with the battalion commander. When the LCP was loaded, it headed for shore, and before long grated on the sand. The front gate was dropped down, and we jumped into waist-deep water and waded ashore.

Once on the shore, I dropped my life belt, quickly assembled my men and struck off inland, following the roads marked by the M.P.'s. The whole scene seemed to be one of utter confusion. Heavily laden soldiers were walking in every direction, trucks roared by, life belts were scattered everywhere and equipment was piled high. The whole thing seemed a hopelessly confused mess to me, as we followed the paths and roads previously cleared of mines and taped off by the engineers. We were most careful to walk between those white tapes, for on all sides of us were mine fields, marked by the Germans with signs bearing the death's head and *Achtung! Minen!* First we crossed the ruined shore defenses, now blasted to bits by the tremendous air and sea bombardment, splashed through the flooded lowlands directly behind the beach and headed inland. Now and then we passed one of our secret seaborne tanks, knocked out by enemy fire in the assault landing. These tanks, equipped with propellers and canvas coverings to float them, must have surprised Jerry.

On we trudged, mile after mile, our heavy, water-soaked clothes adding to our discomfort. Before we reached our assembly area, about 7 miles from where we landed, most of us had suffered severe and painful galling in the groins from our wet clothes. The loads we carried were terrific. In addition to my regular web equipment, I carried a litter and two shell cases loaded with medical equipment. All of my men also were heavily loaded. One boy carried a *full* 5-gallon can of water, another a complete splint set, another a blanket set, others carried litters and medical supplies and so forth. All this was in addition to each man's regular web equipment. By the time we reached our destination, about 1800 hours, we were ready to drop.

The first thing we heard when we arrived in the assembly area was that all plans had been changed. The 4th Division had hit trouble and had not made the progress expected. Consequently, our objectives were changed, and all our briefing and planning on the boat were in vain. What a glum welcome to France that was! At the assembly area I dispersed my men and located Tony. Then I started to dig my first foxhole, and two or three sweating hours later I quit. It wasn't deep enough or long enough or wide enough, but I was too tired to care. I pulled a K ration from one of my pockets, opened it and sat on the edge of my foxhole, eating the cold food and wondering what it would be like up front. In the distance I heard the chatter of machine guns, and closer at hand the roar of our own artillery guns firing. About dusk two Boche planes roared overhead for a bit of strafing, but they were driven off by the heavy .50-caliber fire and by two American planes close behind. Finally, I lay down in my cramped foxhole, wrapped in a shelter-half, my only protection against rain and cold. Of course, it rained that night.

The next day we spent nervously getting ready to go into battle. There really wasn't much to do, but we tried to keep busy. Parachutes of the paratroopers of the 82nd Airborne Division, which had landed on D-Day, were strewn everywhere—in trees, on the hedgerows and in the fields. Here and there were many supply bundles that had been dropped by parachute, but never retrieved. During the morning I went out to find some medical supplies, and located several large bundles of paratroop supplies, untouched. I brought back a few light splints and aluminum folding litters. While on this mission I saw my first dead German soldier. He was a small, young fellow, and he lay behind a stone wall, alone. The bandages on his body showed that he had not been killed instantly, but had died of wounds. During the afternoon our two jeeps and trailers arrived, having just been unloaded from a Liberty ship. We were glad to see them, for now we had all our equipment, and were ready for the battle.

Chapter Five

BAPTISM OF FIRE

On THE EVENING OF FRIDAY, JUNE 9, THE BATTALION commander called the officers together to tell us that we were to march up to the front that night, relieve part of the 82nd Airborne Division, and attack at dawn. About 2300 we got our jeeps ready and "stood by" with our men, waiting for word to pull out. The Heinies were making an air attack on the beach, and over in that direction the sky was ablaze with the brilliant display of .50-caliber tracers and bursting ack-ack shells. I could never describe my mixed emotions or tell just what I thought as I sat there in the darkness watching the "fireworks," listening to the distant sounds of war, and knowing that in a few hours I'd be up there in the thick of battle.

About midnight we got orders to move out, and our long march to the front began. The battalion was strung out in double file, with 5 yards between men. As usual, the medics marched at the rear, and behind us came our jeeps and trailers. It was a pitch-black night, so dark that I had trouble following the man in front of me. On we marched in silence for three hours, through the ruins of St. Mere Eglise, past our own flashing, roaring artillery guns and closer and closer to the enemy. Even today, the memory of that dark night seems like a nightmare.

About 0300 we halted in an advance assembly area, dispersed our men and started to dig foxholes; but in a short time moved out again as the first streaks of daylight appeared, this time for the attack. The day before, a bitter tank and infantry battle had taken place along the road over which we were advancing to the jump-off point for our attack. At one place the road crossed a stream, and the bridge was "zeroed-in" by a Kraut "88,"* which kept slapping in shells smack on the bridge. Quite a few American boys were hit there. We had to cross that bridge, and I realized that the only way to get my men going was to lead them over. I waited until one shell had hit, and then with a "Let's go, boys!" started off down the road and across the bridge at a dog trot, hoping and praying that we'd make it before the next shell landed. We did, and were well away from the bridge when the next round smashed in.

And there I was, in battle. But what confusion! I can't remember any clear-cut facts, but I can never forget the overall picture as I trotted up the road in the eerie half-light of dawn—the mass of milling soldiers, the sharp crack of enemy shells, the stinging odor of cordite on my eyes and nose, the many burned-out tanks strewn along the road and in the fields, and the dead German and American soldiers in great numbers.

But I had other things to think about. A shell cracked down on the road a short distance in front of me, and when I reached that spot I found several boys sprawled on the ground. Two were already dead, one was dying and two were less seriously injured. After quickly looking them over, I left a couple of aid men to bandage the wounds and started up the road again. I had to keep up with my battalion and set up an aid station and try to bring a semblance of order out of this chaos. I had no idea where Tony was or where most of our men were. I had six or eight with me, but the others were scattered.

I was getting desperate; I had to find a spot for an aid station soon, for I knew the casualties would be coming back shortly. I was about to enter the ruins of an old barn, when a passing major shouted, "Keep out of there! It's full of duds!" I hastily backed away. A little farther up the road I came to a group of French farm buildings, and in one wrecked building off the courtyard I set up my

---

* The German 88-mm. gun was an extremely efficient, all-purpose artillery piece, and was hated by all of us.

first station. Our regimental C.P. was in the main farmhouse, and an 82nd Airborne aid station was in the barn. We pushed aside the wreckage in the room to make way for our work, and then I stepped just outside the doorway into the courtyard to look around.

Suddenly there was the sharp, staccato clatter of a German machine pistol, and bullets spattered around me, one of them striking the door frame, not 4 inches from my head. With one mighty leap I was inside the house on the floor. One of the numerous Kraut snipers we encountered in Normandy was in a near-by tree, and had taken a few shots at me. Two or three paratroopers heard the shots, sauntered out with rifles at "ready," and soon shot him out of his tree.

About that time some 88's ripped over the house. That same gun was still shooting at the bridge, each shell passing directly over us and sounding low enough to take off the chimney. Out in front of the farmhouse another German 88 gun had been set up the day before, camouflaged in a clump of trees, to shoot directly down the road. A direct hit by one of our shells had turned the gun over and killed the entire crew. They had been blown into the trees, and now the dead gunners hung limply from the branches, "dripping" down like so much moss. Behind the farmhouse the Germans had defended the position from a long trench. Now it was filled with dead Krauts and the equipment of war strewn everywhere. War is far from pretty.

A few minor casualties came back, but nothing serious. I heard that our battalion's attack was going well, and that the boys had taken the little town of Amfreville and had moved on through it. Tony arrived and our jeeps had come up, so we decided to move on to Amfreville. We piled onto our already heavily loaded jeeps and trailers and drove down the road a mile or two into Amfreville. Oh, what a mess that village was! Our heavy shelling had badly smashed it, and dead soldiers lay crumpled everywhere in the streets. Most were Krauts, but some were our paratroopers.

We looked around for a place to establish an aid station, and finally set it up in a building the Germans had used for a dressing station and had recently evacuated. Behind the building 15 or 20 German soldiers who had been severely wounded and had died were laid out on the ground, the blood forming dark pools beside them. Inside the building on some straw lay a dead body, completely naked except for bandages over a head wound. At first I thought it was a dead Heinie, until I saw the dog tags, and realized that the body was that of a paratrooper whom the enemy had brought in wounded.

Now we began getting more and more casualties from our battalion. We could hear the clatter of a terrific fight up ahead, and we heard that the outfit had hit an enemy strong point. Reports filtered back that sounded none too good.

"They're shooting the hell out of us!"

"Lieutenant Howard has been killed!"

"The Heinies are counterattacking, and will soon retake this town!"

We were busy treating casualties in our station, but we were still uneasy about our position. When we learned that the battalion C.P. had pulled back out of town, we decided we'd better get out, too. By this time the firing was much closer, and had moved around to another side of town, so we were worried about being cut off.

We sent back our last casualties, loaded our men on the vehicles and pulled out of one side of town, just as firing broke out on the opposite side. We moved back a mile or so and reopened our station in an old farmhouse, partially occupied by men of the 82nd Airborne. And now more bad casualties streamed in. About 1800 hours, when we had completed our work, Tony and I were summoned to a battalion commanders' meeting. The officers were told that we would attack again in two hours. Our attack against the enemy strong point that afternoon had failed, so we were to hit it again at 2000 from a different direction after marching around it.

In about 15 minutes the troops rose wearily to their feet, and we started out for the I.P.* We learned that this was to be a regimental attack, with all three battalions in it. On the route we were pestered by enemy snipers who infested the Normandy countryside. Although they hit nobody during that march that I know of, they kept us in an uproar. We hit the dirt frequently, and did a lot of

* The point of departure of an attack.

crawling on hands and knees down these roads while the bullets zinged overhead.

At last we reached the I.P., pulled the jeeps off into a field behind a hedgerow and sat down in a ditch to wait. In our inexperience, we had moved much too far forward for an aid station, and soon we found that out. Lying behind the same hedgerow were the riflemen who were to make the attack. Now our artillery opened up from behind us on the enemy positions, and shells whistled over us. Suddenly it ceased; whistles shrilled, the infantrymen leaped over the hedgerow toward the enemy, and all hell broke loose.

I'd never heard such a racket. Rifles, machine guns, mortars and hand grenades from both sides made a terrific pandemonium. Soon it began to get quite "hot" where I was. Bullets zipped through the trees and mortar shells hit all around. A few dazed soldiers staggered back, saying that the battalion was being cut to pieces.

I couldn't work where I was, so I decided to move back a bit to a more secluded spot. I couldn't find Tony or any of my men; but I started to crawl back myself through a wheat field, while machine gun bullets seemed to clip the top off the grain above me, and enemy mortar shells jarred the earth around me. When I came to a sunken road I jumped into it and sat down to rest a moment, feeling a little safer there.

Down the road came some walking wounded. It was getting dark now, and I had to act quickly and set up an aid station somewhere. I remembered that back up the road about a half mile was a little old French house, so I started for that with my patients. When I reached it I found that already 10 or 12 very badly wounded boys had been brought there and laid on the ground in an adjacent field. I found one medical jeep and two men from the first battalion section there, too, so we went to work. Gradually, the men from the first and third battalion sections appeared. Tony, Jack Gable and Vic di Leo arrived and we moved inside a shed, where we worked all night long. The casualties poured in at an alarming rate, and many of them were bad ones, too. Our litter bearers were having a real workout, bringing in the wounded, and in the aid station we were working at top speed. So heavy were the casualties that we shipped them back to the rear in 2½-ton trucks.

41

By morning most of the wounded had been evacuated, so we thought we'd get a rest; but we were mistaken. Soon after daylight our boys attacked, and attacked again and again all day. It was brutal up there, and what a slaughter! The wounded poured back in dozens, and I've never seen such horrible wounds, before or since— legs off, arms off, faces shot away, eviscerations, chests ripped open and so on. We worked at top speed, hour after hour, until we were too tired to stand up—and then we still kept going. How many lives we saved by the hundreds of units of plasma we gave I'll never know. The first and third battalion aid stations were working together here, so four physicians, two chaplains and all our technicians were working constantly.

It was a bit "hot," too. Machine guns and rifles not far away made quite a din; stray bullets continually whizzed by the aid station, and mortar and 88-mm. shells hit uncomfortably close. During a lull in the stream of casualties Jack Gable and I were standing in the doorway of the station. Suddenly, with an angry crack, an 88-mm. shell hit the chimney of a house across the road. The concussion knocked us back into the station, and fragments of steel whined through the air. We were unhurt, but the leg of a man at an antitank gun farther down the road was almost torn off. We administered first aid and plenty of plasma to him.

Late in the afternoon word came to Tony and me that our battalion was to be pulled out and marched around to attack the strong point from the flank. I have never forgotten the expressions on the faces of those officers as they were again ordered to lead their exhausted, battered companies into another futile, costly assault. Their tired, old-looking, lined, bearded faces, their bloodshot eyes, their torn, muddy clothes, and their grim lips told the story.

A little later the tired, bloody soldiers filed wearily by, and we followed at the rear of the column with our two litter jeeps, equipment and a few men. After traversing a long, circuitous route we stopped in a sunken road, from which the attack was to begin. At a quiet signal, the infantrymen got up and started crawling forward, leaving us unarmed medical personnel sitting there alone in the twilight. We were most uneasy—we didn't know quite where we were, and we didn't know where the Germans were. There was a good bit of danger from snipers, roving enemy patrols and counterattacks.

All was quiet. Then suddenly the Krauts saw our approaching men, and the firing began. Oh, what a fight! Bullets whizzed over as thick as bees, it seemed, while we hugged the ground. We noticed that we had parked our jeeps in an exposed part of the road, where bullets could easily hit them and knock them out—and we couldn't afford that. Tony and I couldn't order our drivers to move those jeeps in that hail of lead, so we both jumped up from our sheltered spot to do it ourselves. We took a jeep apiece, turned them around in record time, and moved them to a place in the road protected by high banks.

Soon the firing slackened a bit, and our litter bearers brought in some wounded. The attack had failed again, we heard. We treated the wounds, loaded about five casualties on each jeep and returned to the aid station. All night long, again, the injured lads poured into our station as the gallant, tireless litter bearers carried them back through the pitch-black woods and fields, from where they had fallen before the German positions. About 0200 the boys brought in Major Ronan, the battalion executive officer, and a friend of mine, shot through the chest. He was cold, pulseless and nearly dead. For an hour I worked by the feeble beams of a flashlight, bandaging his critical wounds and struggling to get a needle into his collapsed veins to give him plasma. My efforts were successful, and when he left the station his condition was fair, and he was talking to me.

So it went for five wild days and nights—attack, attack, attack, again and again and again, with bloody losses each time. During those five days we treated about 150 men a day in the combined first and third battalion aid stations. For five days and nights I did not wash, I did not shave, I did not sleep, except for a rare, brief catnap, and I hardly ate, except to gulp part of a cold K ration when things slowed up now and then. How the litter bearers lasted I do not know. The long litter hauls through that rough hedgerow country were tough. We were all a sight to see, and I must have been the worst. With my blood-caked uniform, my bearded, dirty face, bloodshot eyes and my bloody hands, I was no beauty.

In my memory today, those first few hectic, flaming days of battle seem a hopelessly confused nightmare. Nothing seemed real, and days ran into nights and nights into days without meaning. Time almost stopped, and a week seemed like a month; but always in my mind I can see the never-ending stream of bleeding, dying, mangled boys whom the litter bearers brought in. In a matter of days all of us had become seasoned veterans of battle. Men rose to great heights and proved themselves men, or else went to pieces and revealed themselves as craven souls. Heroic deeds were commonplace, and usually went unnoticed.

Events seem hazy, and are not remembered clearly, but I do have painfully clear memories of watching so many of my friends come through the aid station. I hated to see the fine young infantry officers I had known so well and "buddied" with coming in all shot up. I remember Captain Wheeler Coy (Battalion S-3), limping in with a nasty hole in his heel from a German bullet, frowning disgustedly at having been knocked out of the fight so soon, and looking so tired and worn. I remember Major Jastre (executive officer of the second battalion), gasping for air and turning greenish from a huge sucking chest wound, while I struggled unsuccessfully to save his life. He had rallied his disorganized battalion and had personally led the men in a brilliant counterattack, when a mortar-shell burst riddled him.

I remember Lieutenant Schiller, staggering into the station, holding his bleeding, shattered shoulder. I remember Lieutenant Bowman, lying in a pool of blood in the station, after an 88-mm. shell hit his jeep. I thought he was dead when he was carried in, but he was in good condition when we sent him back to the collecting company. I remember Captain Buck Shaw, when a litter squad carried him in after he had lain seriously wounded all night long in No Man's Land. One of our aid men, Tschabrun, had found him about dark, and had voluntarily stayed all night with him until it was light enough to bring the wounded officer in.

I remember the soldier who had watched with horror and terror as a lumbering tank rolled over his legs as he lay helplessly wounded on the ground. I remember the lad whose entire lower jaw was shot away. I remember the badly wounded boy who was brought in

44

covered with mud and grass after he had lain unnoticed in a ditch for several days.

And I remember so many others, too. Casualties were far too numerous for us to evacuate by ourselves, and many of them were hauled back to us on infantry jeeps or were carried back by comrades on makeshift litters. One bit of mute evidence of the tremendous number of wounded men treated in our station was the huge pile of discarded weapons outside. Before the injured boys came in, their weapons were dropped outside the station, and within a short time there was a large pile of Garand rifles, tommy guns, bayonets, trench knives, Browning automatic rifles, pistols, helmets, packs, blankets and so on. These things represented the less seriously hurt boys, for the stretcher cases usually came in without such equipment. Their weapons were left where they had fallen. Later on, ordnance troops collected this discarded equipment, outside our aid station, but not before the pile had reached staggering proportions. Of course, all around the aid station, inside and out, were scattered great numbers of empty plasma bottles, bloody bandages, torn shoes, blood-soaked parts of uniforms, battered helmets, used morphine syrettes, blood-spattered litters and blankets, splints and so forth.

To the uninitiated, it might seem strange that our division had so many casualties right away, but it is really not so surprising. We were all green, and inexperienced in war, so we did many things wrong. No matter how much soldiers maneuver and train, it takes the real thing to whip them into an efficient fighting force. Before long the 90th Division began to function like a well-oiled machine, but during those first few days all was confusion and error from top to bottom. It is always so in any division when it is first under fire. Then, too, we were facing experienced German soldiers in well-dug-in defenses in this cursed hedgerow country, ideally laid out for defense. It would have been a tough job for combat veterans, but our untried troops were given the task. And so, many men made mistakes and were killed, but those who lived learned quickly by their experience.

On Wednesday, June 14, Tony and I moved our aid station back to Amfreville into a building the Krauts had used for an infirmary.

During the morning we both went to the battalion C.P. "up front," dodging mortar and 88-mm. shells. I had the unpleasant experience of being shot at by a sniper with a machine pistol, but he missed. It's strange how certain pictures stick in your mind. I have seen thousands of dead Germans, but one in particular I remember. He had been killed by a bullet, and had fallen dead on his back in the middle of an open gateway to a field. I saw him frequently during the several days' fighting around Amfreville. No one ever moved him, and everyone walked around him. There he lay, his sightless eyes staring up, his skin getting progressively darker and his abdomen becoming more and more distended. The last time I saw his bloated face, it was purplish black and bulging over his tight collar.

Toward evening I heard that our boys were having trouble evacuating casualties, so I took a litter jeep and two litter squads and went forward. It's not so easy to go forward into a hellhole of death and fear, knowing you may never return, but I could never order my men up there if I were afraid to go. Besides, they needed help and a boost in morale. The morale was zero. Everyone was tired beyond words and discouraged by our failure to advance and by the extremely heavy casualties.

So up we went. Shells dropped around, snipers shot at us, machine guns crackled and bullets popped above us. Of course, I was scared, but I tried to appear calm and to quiet my jittery litter squads. Some of the fellows were as nervous and jumpy as cats. We located the casualties, carried them to where we had left the jeep, and long after dark finally got back to the aid station, where we treated the casualties.

The next day was June 15, my fourth wedding anniversary. I thought about a lot of things that day. I thought about Adrienne, wondered if she knew I was in Normandy, wondered where I'd be on my fifth anniversary or if I'd still be alive, and remembered the beautiful scene of our marriage. I had other things to think about, too. Casualties kept coming in, and so did the enemy fire. During the afternoon I heard that a wounded paratrooper had been hidden from the Germans by a French family in their farmhouse, and now that our lines had been pushed out, we could get to him. I took my jeep and went out to look for him.

I found him up near the front lines, lying calmly and cheerfully in a French farmhouse, with his bandaged leg propped up in front of him. He had an infected bullet wound of his left lower leg, sustained on D-Day, nine days before. He had hidden in the woods until this family found him and took him in. He was in excellent spirits, and seemed not at all worried. He was just like all those magnificent men of the 82nd Airborne Division. No finer fighting men ever lived. They fought with a fury and skill and daring that were an inspiration to all of us. They appeared to be fearless and oblivious to danger. I shall always respect the great American paratrooper.

The glider troops who landed in Normandy on D-Day had a rough time, too. Landing the gliders in that hedgerow terrain was most difficult. There were scores of gliders littering the countryside, many of them wrecked. I saw gliders of which the entire load of passengers had been killed in the crash, and other gliders, the passengers of which had been killed by enemy machine gunners as they stepped from the planes.

While I was getting the injured paratrooper evacuated, I also treated several French people who had been wounded during the fighting. Several wounds were rather bad, and one was critical. The worst wound had been sustained by a pretty girl of about 20 years, who had a week-old chest wound. Now, of course, the wound was badly infected, and she had a high fever. I took her back to the aid station, where I dressed the nasty hole in her chest, gave her plasma and sent her back to our hospitals in the rear. Her condition was extremely poor, and I wonder if she lived.

Late in the afternoon we learned that the 357th and 358th regiments were to jump off at about 2000 in an all-out assault on the little town of Gourbesville and the strong point. Before the attack started, we moved our aid station forward into an old farmhouse, up close to the front. The infantrymen attacked with pent-up fury, and by dark had taken all objectives and routed the Krauts from the strong point. We considered moving our aid station down into

47

Gourbesville after dark, after it was taken, but decided not to. Later we were thankful we had not done so, for the road into that town was mined, and several trucks which passed over it that night were blown up, with considerable casualties.

Just after daybreak a group of German prisoners were marched by, carrying several of their wounded, who were left at our aid station. These were the first wounded German soldiers I had treated, but they were not the last. During the rest of the war I cared for many, many more enemy soldiers, and I always gave them the best care I could.

A little later in the morning Tony and I walked down into Gourbesville, tagging the many American dead in the fields as we went. Some were not pretty sights, especially those who had received close or direct hits by mortar shells. Just outside the town we found the body of Colonel Sheehy, our regimental commanding officer, killed in an ambush two days before, while reconnoitering enemy positions in preparation for the regimental attack.

Since the enemy was still throwing in shells, some too close for comfort, we soon retired from this area. I'll risk my life anytime to help an injured person, but I will not risk it simply to put tags on dead bodies. I am glad the people back home could not see these dead bodies of their loved ones. It is better to think of a neat white cross in a pretty cemetery than the rotting masses of flesh which I saw. Our Graves Registration detail did a good job, but they could not pick up the dead while a battle was raging, and frequently bodies would be missed in bushes, high grass and so forth. Consequently, often a corpse would lie for days or weeks before being picked up. Sometimes heads, arms or legs would be gone, ripped off by shell bursts. The sun and insects did the rest.

Later in the day the enemy fire slackened, and we learned that the Krauts had pulled out from in front of us. We were ordered to pack up, and that evening we marched several miles to an assembly area, where we were to get a couple of days' rest. We spent Saturday and most of Sunday (June 17 and 18) resting and cleaning and mending equipment and writing letters.

We also caught up on the latest news. The 9th and 79th Infantry divisions had now landed and were in action. The 9th was making great progress, and soon would have the peninsula cut in two. We were glad to know that other divisions were coming in behind us. So far we had felt quite "alone." Usually, our flanks were open, and it was a bit uncertain just where the enemy was and where friendly troops were, with respect to the flanks. It was reassuring to know help was coming.

I don't think any of us ever considered the possibility that we couldn't hold the beachhead. After the war I read in Captain Harry Butcher's *My Three Years With Eisenhower* that the high command had figured that we had a 50–50 chance of holding the beachhead, but I'm glad I didn't know that at that time.

Chapter Six

ACROSS THE COTENTIN PENINSULA

SUNDAY AFTERNOON, JUNE 18, WE GOT ORDERS TO move. Our division was to relieve the 9th, which had now reached the western side of the Cotentin Peninsula. We were to block the western side of the peninsula to prevent the enemy from sending any troops up to reinforce Cherbourg and also to keep the Germans from escaping from the Cherbourg trap. The regimental sector was too wide to cover completely, so it consisted of strong defensive areas by each battalion, with thinly held gaps between.

Sunday evening the regiment was moved westward in trucks, and we effected relief of elements of the 9th without trouble. But the next morning, when our third battalion started to push out a little, we hit a hornet's nest. Enemy infantry and a few tanks let the boys come in, and then shot the daylights out of them. For a while it was a rough, confused business. Some of our men were cut off and captured; some were killed and many were wounded.

In the aid station we again had more to do than we could handle. And for a while it was quite "hot" around us, as enemy mortar and 88-mm. shells crashed around the station. An 88 hit a tree not far from the station, literally tearing apart a radio operator beneath it. He was immediately carried to the aid station, but we couldn't help a dead man.

During the height of the action Sergeant Gamble, one of our best aid men, came back to the aid station to ask for some help in evacuating a couple of casualties from a place jeeps could not reach.

He started back with a litter squad of four men, but before they got there they ran into enemy troops and all were captured. Later, Sergeant Gamble and one other of the boys escaped and got back to our lines, after some harrowing experiences. Another, Pfc. Nation, was recaptured at Rennes in Brittany. What happened to the other two I do not know.

Late in the afternoon Major Brown (our regimental surgeon) came down to tell me that he was sending me to take command of the second battalion aid station, which had been having some trouble. I moved there early in the evening, and was with them from then until I left the infantry in October. Ed Rapp, the regimental dental officer, was my assistant at first, and what a swell job he did! I learned that the second battalion had had a very bad time that day, too. One company had pushed out into a swamp, had hit all sorts of trouble, and most of the company had been lost.

I spent the next day getting things organized and getting acquainted. The aid station was in an old French barn, with stone walls about 3 feet thick. It was one of the outbuildings surrounding the courtyard of a château in which was the battalion command post. The battalion was on the line about a mile from us, so I went up to the front to learn the locations of all the companies.

On Thursday, June 22, the battalion attacked in order to get better positions. The enemy resistance was bitter, and the going in that miserable hedgerow country was hard and slow. All day the casualties streamed in, and we were busy every minute. Late in the afternoon we got word that there were three critically wounded men up on the very front line. Twice I sent litter squads to get them, but each time the squads were unable to get through, once because of heavy enemy mortar fire and once because a German machine gun opened up on them. Finally, about dusk, I decided to try to get to the casualties myself. I took three volunteers for litter bearers (I'd make the fourth) and one volunteer jeep driver. I wanted a minimum of men with me, for there was no sense in risking more lives than was necessary. We drove the jeep as far as I thought we dared, and there we left the jeep and driver. Then the three litter bearers and I started out. What a journey! We walked along in darkness, not knowing just where we were, wondering if one of those crashing mortar shells would get us, if one of our own men might shoot us in the dark, and if we'd suddenly blunder into a German position. Finally we located a company command post, and a runner led us to where the wounded lay.

They were really on the front line. They lay on the edge of a field along an old country dirt road. One company was dug in along the road, and across the road, dug-in in the next field, were the Germans. Fire from machine guns and "burp guns" whizzed by, and a few hand grenades exploded here and there. It was no place for us medics, with no foxholes to duck into. And all the while shells from mortars and artillery guns sighed overhead, to rake the roads to the rear, over which we had just come and over which we had to return.

One of the three wounded boys was dead, another had a very severe compound fracture of the skull, and the third had a compound fracture of the leg. The two living casualties we carried back, one at a time, over the dark, fire-swept fields to the road where our jeep awaited us. By now the enemy artillery fire had lifted and was falling on rear installations, but what a mess it had made around here! Trees were all down, the ground was torn up and there were holes in the road.

Miraculously, the jeep had not been knocked out, although it had several holes in it from flying steel; nor had the driver been hurt in his place of refuge under the jeep. We evacuated the casualties to the rear as quickly as we could. Soon after I got back to the aid station the Krauts again began shelling the area around the station, shooting particularly at the crossroads about 200 yards away. The shells rocked the ground and steel fragments bounced off the walls, but no direct hits were scored on our barn.

The next day was moderately busy for us, but it was that night that we had another never-to-be-forgotten thrill and narrow escape. Our second battalion was holding a position a mile or two from where we were located; the third battalion was doing likewise several miles away, and during the afternoon the first battalion moved back into reserve, and dug in about a quarter of a mile from our aid station. That night a desperate group of about 175 German soldiers sneaked down from the north, trying to get through our lines and join the main German army to the south. They crawled down a ravine about 50 yards from the aid station, captured the outpost of the first battalion and suddenly came upon members of the first battalion asleep in their foxholes at about 0330.

Then began a weird, mixed-up fight in the darkness. I awoke to hear a full-scale battle raging just outside the aid station—rifles and pistols cracking, machine guns and "burp guns" chattering, hand grenades exploding, men running and yelling and bullets ricocheting off the stone walls of our barn. There we lay in the darkness in the barn, feeling like rats in a trap. We had no weapons, and how was a Kraut soldier to know we were unarmed medics? Even if he did know, he might kill us, anyway. I kept wondering if a German soldier might not come running by the barn and toss a hand grenade in "for good measure" and wipe us out.

The minutes dragged by so slowly while the battle raged, and we in the aid station lay on the floor, "sweating it out."

Ed Rapp, who was beside me, said in a funny voice, "Mac, is it cold or am I shaking because I'm scared?"

To which I answered, "I don't know, Ed; but I'm shaking, too, and I'm scared!"

About an hour after the fight started it ended, with 150 of the Germans prisoners and the rest killed or injured. Our men suffered about 13 killed and 12 wounded.

It was just getting light now, as the prisoners were being rounded up. We were quite busy again, taking care of about 20 wounded (both American and German) who were all brought to us about the same time. Two company aid men from the first battalion were among those killed. Some of the wounds were very serious, such as those of one of our lieutenants who had compound fractures of both arms and both legs, and who later died.

It was while we were in this location that another of our own aid men was killed: Sergeant Colwell. He was in his foxhole with his company up front, when a mortar shell landed in his foxhole. When a shell hunts a man out like that, he has little chance.

I had thought that after our first two weeks in battle, when our casualties were so heavy, the 90th Division was too badly mauled to function well, and that it might have to be sent back to England to be reorganized. That was only my idea, and it was far from the plan in this war. As a division suffered losses, replacements were sent up and the units went on fightting as before. We received many replacements during the Normandy campaign, some of whom were killed on the way up, before they reached their new assignments. Not infrequently new men who did come up were killed before they had met their officers or buddies. Life in Normandy in those days was confused and precarious.

And so the days went by, in the Portbail area. Each night the Krauts would shell the crossroads a couple of hundred yards from us, sometimes using only one gun and sometimes using several. Once in a while the shells landed dangerously close to our station, but they never hit it directly. We had to drive over this crossroads in our jeeps to get to the battalion to evacuate casualties; so we'd wait in front of the station until a shell landed, and then take off like a flash and race around the corner, "hell bent for election," before the next shell came in. By doing that, none of us was ever hit there.

One night, however, we had an especially heavy shelling. There were a lot of close hits, but I kept telling myself that we were fairly safe in the aid station, with the thick stone walls around us (although I really didn't feel at all safe). I would have felt much worse had I known that all night there was a truck loaded with ammunition parked right beside our barn. When I saw it there in the morning, I lost no time in having it moved.

For about 10 days we remained here, and then we pulled out. Cherbourg had fallen, and the northern part of the Cotentin Peninsula had been cleaned out. Elements of the 79th Division relieved our regiment, and we took a 2-day rest before starting the next phase. I remember the day we pulled back for the rest because of the bad weather. I had no raincoat yet, and a cold rain soaked me through and through that afternoon. I spent a miserable night lying on the muddy ground, protected from the pelting rain only by a soggy blanket.

One cannot really describe the discomfort of the infantry in bad weather; one has to feel it oneself to be able to understand it. Imagine a 10-mile march in a pouring rain, during which men and equipment are soaked through, and meals consist of cold cans of chopped ham and eggs and some soggy crackers. Then contact is made with the enemy, and the men quickly deploy into battle positions. They crawl toward the enemy through mud and tangled underbrush, while shells and bullets scream overhead. Some of their buddies are killed. Toward dark the attack halts, and the men dig foxholes in the sloppy ground. When the holes are big enough and deep enough, the boys climb into them, cursing the pelting rain as it puddles in their foxholes. During the night they sit in their cramped quarters, cold, hungry and soaking wet. Enemy artillery intermittently hammers the area, and several times during the night the weary boys must fight hard to beat off savage German counterattacks. At dawn they again begin a bloody, muddy advance, and this continues day after day for endless, nameless month after month.

At about this point our morale reached a low ebb. We were dazed by the shattering battles of the preceding weeks and by the wholesale slaughter and mangling of so many comrades. We were tired and dirty and uncomfortable, and we could see no end to this miserable existence. If we were going to have to keep on battling our way yard by yard clear to Berlin, it would take us a decade.

And then the electrifying news spread through the ranks like wildfire that General Patton was in Normandy. All sorts of quotations said to have been his words were repeated over and over.

"Patton says he'll be in Paris in a month."

"Patton says he can break out of Normandy any time now."

"Patton says he'll be in Berlin in 90 days."

How many of these declarations he actually made I don't know; but the fact that "Old Blood and Guts" was here, breathing out fire and brimstone and ready to tear into the Krauts, gave all of us a boost. The pros and cons of his character have been debated hotly, but the fact remains that his mere presence inspired troops with confidence and optimism. In those dark Normandy days the soldiers seemed to think: "'Blood and Guts' is here. Now we'll go places. Let his tanks roll!"

But we had a long way to go yet—farther than any of us thought.

Chapter Seven

HILL 122 AND BEYOND

*A*FEW DAYS LATER, ON JULY 3, THE 90TH DIVISION began its historic and bloody assault on the heavily fortified enemy positions in the Forêt de Monte Castre, better known to us as "Hill 122." The positions were defended by crack troops, who elected to stay and fight and die, rather than to retreat. For the first couple of days the 357th Regiment was in reserve, but we moved up close to the front and dug in before the attack began, in order to be readily available if needed.

About dawn on July 3 the awe-inspiring preättack artillery barrage began. The ground trembled and shook from the roar of big guns, as I lay in my foxhole in the rain wondering when we'd be thrown into the battle. Reports filtered back to us about the bitter fighting going on, and about the extremely heavy casualties the other two regiments were sustaining.

Late that afternoon the battalion moved around to a different location, still very close to the fighting. We had all our aid station personnel in an orchard, and there we dug in under fire. Machine guns rattled over the next hill, burp guns ripped too close for comfort, stray bullets sighed by, mortar shells crumped in the next field and 88's peppered the road in front of us. We dug foxholes fast that evening, so we could stay alive in that rain of death.

The next day was the Fourth of July, but it was no holiday. We stayed in our foxholes most of the day, of necessity. The other two battalions of our regiment were committed this day; but we were held in division reserve. The next morning our area was heavily shelled. During the shelling I heard several rounds land in the next field over, and the cry of "Medics!"

I grabbed my aid kit, jumped from my foxhole and ran to the next field, hitting the ground several times on the way as more shells slapped in. When I arrived I found the dead body of a boy in headquarters company, whom I had known and liked, lying in his foxhole. He had been running for the foxhole when a shell hit a few feet from him. Even as he leaped for the safety of the fox- hole a steel fragment ripped through his skull, and his nearly head- less body flopped into the bottom of the hole. I took one look and ran back for my own shelter.

Later in the day it rained, and of course we moved. About dark I learned about our precarious situation as I stood in the rain, mis- erably wet, while shells from a gun battery not far behind us ripped across the sky above us. Things were rather desperate. On our right the two other regiments had been stopped cold on the bloody slopes of Hill 122. In front of us the first and third battal- ions of our regiment had attacked on a narrow front between two swamps, had been stopped and split up, and were being chopped to bits. Now the Germans were launching a vicious counterat- tack between the swamps to annihilate the regiment and break out behind our lines. If they did break through, our battalion would be the only force available to stop them, and we were to hold them at any cost. I did not sleep well in my muddy foxhole, with the rain pouring down on me, the roar of the guns shaking the ground, and my mind wondering when we'd be ordered to the attack or when the enemy might suddenly break through on us in the darkness.

Well, the first and third battalions, although badly cut up, fought magnificently and held the enemy counterattack. It would be impossible to single out any one man or any few men as having stopped the Germans. Every man who stood there and fought deserves the credit. And yet one man, Captain Woodrow Allen, was the inspiration of his men and a rock in the storm. He com- manded K Company of the third battalion. I knew him well and liked him, but I never appreciated his greatness until I saw him in battle. During those early days in Normandy he was a splendid example to all of us. I remember the last time I saw him alive. He was sitting in his foxhole during a lull in the fighting, working over his maps. His dirty, unshaven face looked so tired and lined and worn.

A few days later he led his company down between the swamps and into a furious storm of death. When the enemy counterattack split up the two battalions and cut off the rifle companies from the command posts, he rallied and organized the remnants and held on grimly against smashing enemy attacks. German infantry stormed the positions and German tanks broke through and roamed around behind the defenders, shooting and crushing many. Seventeen times in 24 hours the Krauts threw everything they had at the stubborn force, but Captain Allen and what remained of the two battalions held on. This brilliant defense saved the day, and soon relief came through to rescue the force. A short time after help reached them Captain Allen was killed by a mortar shell, before he could know that his great defense had earned him a battlefield promotion to the grade of major.

Meanwhile, the other two regiments on our right were having a tremendous battle for the possession of Hill 122. It was tough going on the steep slopes, with the heavy, dark forests and tangled underbrush making communication and orientation difficult. At one time, while the third battalion of the 358th regiment was engaged in heavy fighting, the battalion commander, Lieutenant Colonel Bealke, realized that he was lost. He could not determine his position on his maps, hemmed in as he was by the dense forest. He sent a radio message to the 344th field artillery battalion, which was in direct support of his battalion, to help him locate his position. One of the field guns then fired smoke shells fused to burst in the air, toward the colonel's position. Colonel Bealke adjusted the fire of the smoke shells until they were bursting right above him. Then, by consulting maps and firing tables, the artillery officers were able to give the battalion commander his exact location.

The next day our battalion (still in reserve) moved forward and I moved the aid station into a house in the badly damaged town of St. Jores. Since we were in reserve, our casualties were light, but

59

not far away was the roar of battle, and not a few shells came our way. It didn't really start until night, however. About midnight, soon after we had lain down on the floor to sleep, I heard the report of an enemy gun and in a few seconds the crack of the shell exploding not far away. Then another report and another shell—closer. And then another report—and wham! Dust and glass flew as a concussion wave hit us. A shell had landed just outside the house, putting 35 holes in the ambulance, smashing the windows of the house, knocking in part of the wall and spraying lethal steel fragments across the rooms.

For a few seconds we were stunned; then we jumped up to see who had been hurt. Luckily, since we were all lying on the floor, only three men were hurt, but only slightly, by flying glass. Another shell came in, but it zipped directly over the house and landed farther up in town. And so the shelling continued until daylight. The room I was in faced the side from which the shells came, so we sought shelter in a thick-walled wine cellar on the other side of the house. There we spent the night. Many more shells landed close, but none quite as close as before.

One of the worst things about battle is the terrible noise. The angry scream and crack of shells, the roar of artillery, the chatter of rifles and machine guns and the clank of tanks were nerve-wracking. It was surprising, however, how soon we became used to the noise and how quickly we learned the sound of the various weapons. Before long I knew the distinctive "burp" of the Jerry machine pistol, and could tell in a second whether machine-gun fire was ours or the enemy's. The fire of our rifles and BAR's also was quite distinctive.

Sometimes at night, when things were relatively quiet except for shelling by enemy howitzers, we could hear the Heinie guns fire and then, many seconds later, hear the scream of approaching shells. I could always tell by the sound of the guns when they fired, long before the shells arrived, whether or not the rounds would land close to me. If the distant sounds were dull and muffled, the shells would land some distance from me, but if the sounds were clear and sharp, I braced myself for a close one.

The matter of cowardice usually is glossed over by most people who write about soldiers, yet the American army had its share of cowards. These caused some trouble, but usually were not numerous enough to constitute a serious menace.

After the battle between the swamps, Colonel Barth, the regimental commander, called the officers of the second battalion together. He told us that the first and third battalions were exhausted and had been very badly battered. The only effective fighting force in the regiment at the moment was the second battalion. He said that in the other two battalions there had been too many cowards, most of whom were replacements who had been sent up recently. When the going got hot they ran, thus leaving their veteran comrades in trouble, and causing the officers and noncommissioned officers to expose themselves unnecessarily in order to hold the ground. As a result, many fine leaders had been needlessly killed. The colonel said that any man running away thereafter must be shot on the spot. Although I never saw a man shot for cowardice, I understand that such did occur occasionally. However, more than once I have seen an officer pull his gun on one of these cowards and force him back into the fight.

Another unsavory feature was the self-inflicted wound. Frequently a man would wound himself in order to get out of the hell of battle. Although we could seldom prove it, we battalion surgeons could nearly always detect the "S.I.W's." The wound almost invariably was in the hand or foot; there was occasionally a powder burn on the skin, and often the path taken by the bullet was in a difficult angle for it to have come from the direction of the enemy.

The real give-away, however, was the way in which the wounded man acted. A soldier with a bona fide injury would be quiet and stoical, gritting his teeth and seldom moaning in pain. In contrast, the man who had shot himself would put on an act in the way in which he thought a wounded soldier should act. He would shout in pain, call for morphine, sometimes roll around wildly and proclaim how much he hated to have to leave the fight and brag about his prowess at killing Germans.

These self-inflicted wounds were more numerous than one likes to think. They usually came in bunches, occurring most often when the fighting had stalemated temporarily. Many of these men were court-martialed, but few were convicted, for generally there were no witnesses to the deed. Any man shot through the hand or foot was carefully scrutinized and frequently court-martialed, since very few battle injuries were gun-shot wounds of the hand or foot.

I have nothing but contempt for such cowards, although most of us in battle longed for a way out. A nonfatal wound which would not cause permanent disability would be welcome. At least, it would take a man out of this hell for a while and would be the only sure way of not going back dead.

It was during our few days in St. Jores that I took my first "bath" in six weeks. It wasn't much—only pouring cold water over myself—but at least I stood in a real bathtub to do it. The house we were in had one of the few bathtubs I saw in France.

During these battles I treated hundreds of wounded soldiers and I saw many incredible things. Here I might mention three of the cases that stand out in my mind.

The first concerned a young tank officer, a second lieutenant. When his tank had been knocked out by an 88 during the fighting for Hill 122, one of his feet had been virtually torn off. He had pulled himself out of his disabled tank, and a passing aid man had stopped the bleeding and bandaged the wound. Then an enemy counterattack threw back the Americans, so for two days the wounded man lay out there in No Man's Land. During the seesaw fighting back and forth many shells fell near him, and one large piece of steel shattered his other foot. The young fellow pulled off his belt and applied a tourniquet to the leg.

Later, when one of my litter squads found him and brought him in and I heard the story, I expected to see a moribund patient, but such was not the case. He was calm, cheerful and not in shock. In fact, he was in excellent general condition, although both feet hung in tatters and would have to be amputated.

When I remarked to him that he was in surprisingly good condition, he smiled and said, "Well, Doc, I just had the will to live!"

In the second case a 19-year-old boy was wounded on patrol one night. He was the leading scout of a small patrol which ran into some heavy enemy machine-gun fire, and he fell with a compound fracture of the femur (thigh bone). He knew no one could find him in the darkness, so he crawled a half-mile back to his own lines. Don't ask me how he crawled on a broken femur, but he did, and he was not in shock when he arrived at the aid station some time later. He said he needed no morphine, but I gave him some before I splinted his leg.

"Is the chaplain here?" he asked.

Then, as Captain Ralph Glenn, the Protestant chaplain with our battalion, stepped forward, the boy said, "Chaplain, I know that God spared my life out there tonight. Won't you please read from the Bible to me?"

So, as I worked, Chaplain Glenn read to the lad.

The third is a dog story. One evening a soldier was shot in the shoulder, so he started to walk back to the rear to the aid station, but he became lost in the darkness. Finally he crawled into an abandoned foxhole to wait for morning. A short time later he heard a noise and was ready to shoot, when he saw that the noise was made by a little dog. The friendly mongrel jumped into the foxhole and curled up beside the boy, where he stayed all night long.

The next morning, after daylight, the soldier started off again in what he thought was the right direction, but the little dog tugged at his legs and made quite a scene, apparently trying to get the boy to go in the opposite direction. This the boy finally did. As it turned out, the dog led him back to the American lines. Had he kept on in the direction he had selected, he would have walked into the German lines, to death or some wretched prison camp.

After we had dressed the soldier's wounded shoulder and laid him on a stretcher, the little dog jumped up on the boy's abdomen, lay down and would not leave. Since the soldier had formed a strong attachment for his benefactor and did not want to leave him, we loaded the stretcher—soldier, dog and all—into the ambulance and sent them on their way to the hospital.

Before we had been in combat long, we in the aid station formed a high regard for the protection afforded the head by our steel helmet. We saw so many instances in which the helmet deflected shell fragments or ricocheting bullets, or in which the helmet slowed the force of a steel fragment so that instead of a fatal wound's being inflicted only a superficial injury resulted. As one would expect, we were careful to wear our helmets almost all the time.

There are many hazardous and harrowing duties in the infantry, and one of these in particular is patrolling. Nearly every night small bands of men (usually two to four or five) would slip behind the enemy lines to find out all they could about enemy troop movements, plans, disposition of guns and so forth. One can easily imagine what a dangerous, nerve-wracking task this was. Frequently these men never returned, but more often than not they got back. The information they would get often was of great value. Most of the men sent out on patrols at night were simply assigned in rotation, but there were some men who seemed to enjoy such added dangers and who volunteered for patrols. I remember two such men who were sergeants in my battalion. They were experts at this grim game, and went out time after time. Finally, as is usually the case with good infantrymen, one was killed and the other was very seriously wounded.

In a couple of days we moved again. The 358th and 359th regiments were now making slow progress, but the 357th was still "hung up" between the swamps. The mission of our battalion was to move to the right around the right swamp and attack the enemy on the flank. We expected it to be a desperate fight, but when we attacked early in the morning we found that the Krauts had pulled out the night before, leaving only a covering shell. The whole front moved rapidly forward for several miles until we hit the next enemy positions.

As I drove across Hill 122 and through the Forêt de Monte Castre I marvelled that the troops had ever driven the Krauts out. The steep, rugged, rocky slopes, the heavy forests and the excellent natural and prepared defenses made this a wonderful fortress. Our artillery had torn up the area to a terrific degree. Shattered trees, wrecked tanks and guns and huge craters in the roads and fields made the region a shambles. There were many battered bodies of dead Heinies all over the place, too.

I had been shown on a map the new location of the battalion command post, so Ed Rapp and I took a jeep and driver and started out to find it. While passing through the ruins of the little village of Les Plessis, I was stopped by an aid man who asked me to see what I could do for a demented French woman who he thought had gone insane from the heavy fighting. I was irritated by this, because I was in a hurry, but nevertheless we stopped and I went into the house to see what I could do.

Was it Providence that made me stop? At the very moment when I would have been at a road crossing a couple of hundred yards down the road—had I not stopped—seven shells from an enemy 88 slapped in in quick succession, all hitting smack on the corner and causing casualties. I probably owe my life to a "crazy" French woman.

Before we had been long in battle, those of us who still survived had evolved our own philosophy. It was impossible to see our friends and comrades cut down all around us while we remained unhurt, without feeling the presence of a Power far greater than ourselves. We felt that the Lord must be at our sides.

We proceeded on, found the battalion command post and sent back for our men and aid-station equipment. Then we dug our fox-holes, under fire again. Random mortar and 88-mm. shells were coming in quite frequently all around, and stray bullets sighed past us. After I had dug my foxhole I drove back to establish contact with the collecting company. Captain Spicer and Lieutenant Engel decided to accompany me to my aid station to see where it was, so we set out in Spicer's jeep. We were driving down the main road toward Periers at a good clip, and somehow I missed the turn off to the aid station.

On we drove until we were out of our own lines and a couple of miles behind the enemy lines. The first we knew of it was when we rounded a curve and came smack upon an enemy antitank gun fac-ing us a little distance down the road, camouflaged with branches and all ready to fire. On our right in a field were a dozen or so German soldiers, digging foxholes. On our left five or six others were eating supper, and a hundred yards or so behind us a little Kraut was sitting in the ditch beside the road, eating his supper, with his helmet off and his feet up.

The jeep driver jammed on his brakes and threw the jeep into reverse. Why the enemy didn't kill or at least capture us I'll never know. Perhaps it was because of the Red Cross flag on the jeep or perhaps it was because they were as surprised as we were. At any rate, we roared up the road backward at top speed for a mile before we turned the jeep around and sped back to our own lines. I felt more than a little shaky after that close escape. That night the enemy shelled our positions, inflicting casualties, but Ed Rapp and I were not hit in our double foxhole.

The next day we attacked again, made good progress and in a couple of days had pushed to the Seves River, where we held up for a while. I had my aid station for the first few days there in a beautiful, big, heavy stone-walled château just outside the village of Gonfreville. I suppose the enemy thought that such an imposing building must certainly be a command post, for one night they shelled us from dusk to dawn with battery volleys from 100 and 150-mm. guns. Actually, we were not in much danger because the massive walls of our building were good protection, but it was a bit hard on the nerves to lie there on the floor all night long and hear the shells crack down. Some were over, some were short and some hit directly on the house. One direct hit got the ambulance, parked beside the house, and destroyed it. We could hear the guns go off far away; in a few seconds we'd hear the screaming shells coming closer, closer, closer, and then we'd brace ourselves for the concussion. When one would hit the château, the dust would fly and steel fragments would whine through the air. After this experience we moved out into a field the next day and dug foxholes for ourselves.

It was here that the 358th Infantry made its ill-fated and tragic attack on "the Island" in an effort to straighten the lines. "The Island" was a fortified bit of ground in the middle of the swampy Seves River. To get to it, one had to wade through an open, waist-deep swamp about a half-mile wide. Two battalions began the attack soon after daylight. The enemy let our boys come on and then blasted them with all the fury of hell. Dead and wounded disappeared in the swamp as the withering fire cut down the attackers. Those who did reach the island were killed or captured, including one battalion commander and his staff. A few dazed survivors straggled back, but the attack cost the regiment almost one whole battalion and part of another. I thanked God that our regiment had not been called on for that nasty job, or I might now be buried in a French swamp.

It was here that three chaplains of the regiment did a wonderful and courageous deed. After the attack collapsed, many of our wounded men lay helplessly in places too close to the German positions to be reached. The chaplains walked out in full view of the enemy, carrying a white flag of truce. Then they proceeded to pick up all the wounded soldiers they could find and to bring them back. For several hours they worked directly in front of the enemy, but no shots were fired at them.

For about 10 days we sat on the north side of the Seves River, under constant enemy shell fire. Some of it was quite heavy, and we sustained several casualties. A few shells hit very close to me, but again I luckily escaped injury. Then, on July 25, came the American 3,000-plane raid and the beginning of our breakout of Normandy.

I watched the air show from Gonfreville, and what a show it was! First, fighters and fast, low-level bombers roared in to bomb and strafe enemy positions, and then came the fleets of high-flying Liberators and Fortresses—hundreds of them. On they came, flight after flight, seemingly sailing lazily along in perfect formation. Bombs cascaded down and the earth trembled, although I was miles away from where they landed. Flak dotted the sky around the ships, and now and then one of the big planes went spinning down in flames. When this happened we held our breath as we counted the number of white blossoming parachutes, and too often only five or six appeared. When the attack first began the anti-aircraft fire was intense, but it soon lessened as the carpet bombing knocked out gun after gun, and toward the end there was no flak at all, so that the later waves of planes bombed at will.

To the south the big drive for Coutances was on, and now it was time for us to put on our drive to take Periers. That afternoon the 357th Infantry moved to an assembly area on the left for the jump-off the next day. We were to attack southwest on the enemy flank

67

between and in conjunction with the 83rd Infantry and the 4th Armored Division, behind the "Island," while the other two regiments of our division attacked frontally from the north.

I had selected an old farmhouse for my aid station, so we moved into it before daybreak while the soldiers were quietly getting set to storm the enemy lines. At 0400 they hopped off in a surprise attack without artillery preparation. In a matter of seconds the fight was on. I'll never forget the brilliant display I saw from my aid station, as thousands of tracer bullets from the hammering machine guns of both sides streaked across the dawn sky. That was the beginning of a rough day for us. The enemy resistance was fanatical, and after a full day of bitter fighting we had advanced only 300 yards.

Casualties were heavy and bad, and all of us in the aid station were exhausted by the continual stream of wounded. We had more than the usual number of men with combat exhaustion, too—those pitiful men who sit rigidly in the station shaking and crying, with faces and wide eyes filled with horror. We caught more than the usual amount of fire around the aid station that day. Stray bullets made a constant hum, while mortar and artillery shells hit all over the place. We seemed to be charmed, for although there were many close hits, our ruined farmhouse was never struck directly. Across the road from us and behind our house men were being killed and wounded by the heavy shell fire, but we were spared.

Behind the aid station were two knocked-out American tanks, hit by enemy 88's during an attack here several days before. Hanging halfway out of the turret of each tank was the badly burned body of the tanker. When the tanks were disabled the boys had tried to escape from the flaming wrecks, but German bullets had cut them down almost before they could get started. Now the hot summer sun had added much to the sickening sight. Since all our battalion's men passed right by here on their way to the battle, it did not help their morale, so it was my duty to remove the bodies and put them out of sight until the Graves Registration detail could collect them. I did not enjoy that job. We did not look inside the tanks.

It was during this day that I felt myself slipping. I thought I couldn't stand to see many more bleeding, mutilated American boys, to see and smell the rotting bodies of the dead, to hear and cringe under the crash of shells and to see the screaming men with combat exhaustion. I had to get a hold on myself that day to keep going. Whether I might have become a victim of battle exhaustion myself had this kept up I do not know, but the next day the enemy collapsed in front of us and our race across France soon began.

That night, under the cover of a thunderous artillery barrage, the Germans pulled out. All night we lay in the station hearing the shells crash around us, wondering if any of us had a chance to live through this war. About 0300 the barrage ceased, and when the infantry attacked at dawn they found the enemy gone. All that day and the next we pushed rapidly south, capturing Periers and hitting only scattered enemy resistance until we finally met the 1st Division, which had moved west from around St. Lo. Although the enemy resistance was light, our advance was not without casualties, for the Germans had left mines behind.

Periers was full of mines and booby traps, and many roads were mined. One of the jeeps from battalion headquarters was blown up, killing one man and injuring three. The worst hurt of the three was a fine young lieutenant, a friend of mine. He had a compound fracture of one leg, a crushing of the other foot, multiple fractures of his facial bones, severe lacerations of arms and face and a bad concussion. He was covered with dirt and black powder. His wounds were hard to dress.

After we met the 1st Division we stopped for a four-day rest. We did not know, as we took it easy here, that the Normandy campaign was over. It had been long, costly and bloody, and it had been difficult fighting in the jungles of the Normandy hedgerows. These hedgerows were not the prim, low hedges of England, but were formidable obstacles which occurred about every 100 yards, dividing the countryside into square fields. The hedgerows were mounds of earth 4 to 6 feet high, on which grew large trees, bushes, brambles and the like. The Germans had forbidden the French farmers to trim the bushes, so the mounds were overgrown by a thick, tangled mass of shrubs. Such country as this made excellent natural defenses for the enemy, who had added many dug-in strong points, had carefully worked out a plan of defense for the hedgerows and had driven long poles into any large open spaces to prevent gliders from landing. It was a tough nut to crack.

In Normandy, as in the rest of the campaign, it was the infantry company aid men who were the greatest heroes, in my opinion. I do not mean to detract from the glory due the great rifleman, but that aid man shared the same dangers and hardships as the rifleman without the protection of a gun. When the fire was heaviest and everyone else was hugging the ground, the aid man was up exposing himself as he crawled to help those who had been wounded. The tales of the heroism of the aid men were legend. The men they served loved them like brothers. How they managed to put on such good dressings as they lay flat on the ground working on the wounded while bullets crackled overhead and shells exploded on all sides, I'll never know. Many of these gallant lads were killed and many more wounded. They are the real heroes of the war, for my money.

Before D-Day we all had been somewhat concerned about the possible danger from "Bouncing Betty," the antipersonnel mine which the Jerries had used so effectively in Africa and Italy. The "Bouncing Betty" was a steel mine about the size of a flowerpot, buried close to the surface of the ground. When a man stepped on the firing trigger, a small charge of powder would blow the mine into the air after he had taken a few more steps. When the mine reached a height of about 5 feet it would explode, hurling hundreds of steel fragments in all directions. Fortunately, we encountered few of these in France or Germany.

Dead cows were common sights in Normandy, and soon became trademarks of the place to us. Since Normandy is a dairying area, there had been many cows on the farms. Great numbers were killed by shellfire during the fighting, and their bloated, stiff-legged carcasses dotted the fields, not adding to the fragrance or beauty of the land.

Chapter Eight

THE DASH ACROSS FRANCE

*A*FTER OUR REST WE MOVED SOUTH THROUGH Coutances and Averanches to the base of the peninsula near Mortain, where we took up defensive positions for a few days. While we were there I had severe gastroenteritis. I began to feel a little sick late one evening after a cold, greasy supper and by the time I had my foxhole dug I felt sick enough to die. Soon after dark enemy planes appeared overhead and began to bomb in our vicinity. I suppose it was a rather terrifying night, with Jerry bombers flying low over us and our ack-ack lighting the sky with fire, but I was too sick to care. I vomited a few times toward morning and then felt a little better. The next day I went back to the regimental aid station and spent the day there lying on a litter. By the next morning I was able to return to my men, although I felt weak for several days.

It was here at Mortain that the Krauts launched their desperate and violent counterattack in an attempt to cut the American troops off at Averanches, but that happened after we had left. Now the Germans were disorganized and our armored divisions were on the loose. Then the 90th got orders to take off; to strike out boldly to capture Le Mans, far to the southeast. We were just to keep going, not worrying about enemy troops on the flanks and behind us. Just keep going! The plan was to swing a trap around the German 7th Army vainly attacking at Mortain.

Thus began a strange and weird type of warfare. From that time until we ran out of gasoline at Metz it was a race of long spearheads across France. We never knew where the Krauts were, how many there were or what we'd run into. We simply kept smashing ahead. It was all very confusing, but the Germans were more confused than we were. All around us were isolated bands of disorganized Heinies, some of whom chose to fight it out.

The 357th spearheaded the drive to Le Mans. The regiment was motorized, and started out early in the morning of August 5, led by some of the tanks of the 712th Tank Battalion (the 90th Division's attached armor). By late afternoon we had reached Mayenne, which we took that night after a sharp fight. While the first and third battalions attacked frontally the second slipped across the river above the city in rubber assault boats and came in from the side. I took a few litter bearers and aid station men and a small amount of equipment and followed the battalion across. The majority of our men and equipment were to go into Mayenne across the bridge after the town had been taken.

My boat was the last one to cross, and by the time I landed on the far shore all the troops ahead of us had vanished. I set off up a hill over a path through a woods, with six or eight men behind me, not sure where I was or where I was going. I hoped I'd find our own troops soon and not the Germans. I admit I was in a bit of a cold sweat. At last I came out into the open onto a road and found some of the battalion officers with a few of their men. We started walking down the road toward Mayenne, wondering when we'd hit the Germans. To our right an enemy gun was firing across the river and to our left and front there was rifle and machine-gun fire. We were quite confused, but since it was getting dark we wanted to get to Mayenne soon.

Just about dusk we entered the edge of the town, finding our troops already there. I set up an aid station in a small barn near the building in which the battalion command post was located, and waited for the rest of the medical personnel and equipment to arrive. They crossed the river on a bridge in town as soon as it had been taken. Very soon we were ready for work.

Sporadic firing came from the center of the town and from the northeast. It was completely dark by this time and things were still in a confused state. The German commanders in this area did not know we had driven this wedge out from Normandy clear to Mayenne, and had sent small reconnaissance parties to Mayenne to set up a defense there. The main body of troops were to follow the next day.

About an hour after dark a German staff car with three officers (one a medical officer) drove right into the center of town without realizing that it was held by the Americans. When they discovered this and leaped from the car, a burst from a .50-caliber machine gun instantly killed two of the officers and cut the car to pieces. Miraculously, the medical officer was not hit, and he was brought to the command post near my aid station. He knew a little English and I knew a little German and so we were able to converse a bit. It seemed strange to be sitting outside in the dark in a French town talking with a German physician, while the sounds of fighting echoed around us and low-flying planes growled by in the inky sky above. I thought that by the sound of their engines some of the planes might be German, but my companion assured me that they were British. He ought to have known. Soon our troops were in full possession of the town; the rest of the night was quiet.

Late the next day we were relieved by elements of the 9th Division, and we started on the next lap to Le Mans. As we were leaving Mayenne we heard rather heavy firing to our left rear. It made me a bit uneasy to be pushing ahead while enemy troops were behind us, but we left them to the 9th Division. As a matter of fact, members of the 9th Division had a full-scale battle on their hands for the next several days. The strong enemy force which was supposed to have arrived in Mayenne before we did—to defend it against the Americans—appeared shortly after we left it. This force tried desperately to retake the city and to cut our line of communication, but the 9th Division could not be cracked.

Oblivious to this impending fight behind us, we rolled along on the way to Le Mans. The first battalion was in the lead and our second battalion was close behind. Now that we were out in the open and really moving, we were greeted everywhere by throngs of hysterical, cheering French people. How happy they were to see us!

Before long it became dark, and the speed of the long convoy slowed down a good bit. Since a full moon shone down from above, it was not too difficut to see. In a little while the convoy stopped, and we sat there in the summer quiet, wondering what was going on. We knew Germans were all around us, but we hoped there weren't too many.

Suddenly a brilliant flash of orange flame shot up to my left a mile or so away, followed by the dull rumble of a mighty explosion. Then all was darkness and quiet again. I never knew what it was—perhaps the French underground was blowing up an enemy ammunition dump—but it gave me an eerie feeling. Soon enemy planes began to be heard in the sky, flying back and forth. Their pilots had no idea our columns had penetrated so far, and so they were not looking for us there. In spite of the bright moon they could not see us as long as our vehicles did not move. We were under strict orders not to move when the planes were overhead and not to fire at them. As a result, they never discovered us. Had some zealous Kraut pilot dropped some flares and found our convoys, enemy planes could have done tremendous damage, for jeeps, trucks, tanks, big guns, supply trucks and so forth were packed bumper to bumper for a couple of miles.

Word came back to me that there were casualties up ahead, so I took the ambulance directly behind my litter jeep and started up the road past the parked vehicles ahead of us. When I got to the head of the column I found why I had been called. A jeep from regimental headquarters, bearing a captain, a warrant officer and two enlisted men had been ambushed while it had been traveling from the front of our column to the rear of the first battalion some miles ahead. While they were driving along alone on the road the first battalion recently had traversed, they were fired upon by a German patrol which probably had lain in hiding as our vanguards went by. The driver was killed, the jeep was wrecked and the other three men were wounded, the warrant officer and enlisted man seriously. After the ambush the Germans walked out and took the captain with them, leaving the others there for dead. Later, a patrol from our battalion found the two wounded men a short distance ahead of the place where we had stopped. A guide took me and my ambulance to the spot. In the darkness without a light I bandaged the wounds of the two injured soldiers, loaded them into the ambulance, covered the body of the dead man with a blanket and came on back with my escort. The jeep was left there, but in the morning it was gone. Apparently, the German patrol had still been lurking close by, watching us, and after we had gone back to our own troops, had driven off the jeep.

About midnight we were ordered to get our vehicles off the road for the night. I arranged our jeeps and trailers and the ambulance in a field, dispersed the men and then lay down on the ground for a sleep before dawn. Since we were in the same field as a battery of 155-mm. howitzers, I hoped the Luftwaffe wouldn't attack, for those guns would offer a fine target.

In the morning we pushed on to aid the first battalion, which had been having serious trouble up ahead around St. Suzanne. They had gone into and on past the town, but had been attacked from the rear by about 500 fanatical, screaming paratroopers. They had fought a wild pitched battle in the darkness all night. In the streets of St. Suzanne American and German soldiers had fired at each other from point-blank range. The battalion command post in the cellar of one of the buildings had been isolated and attacked by the enemy, so that everyone from the colonel on down fought madly to beat off the foe.

When our battalion arrived it attacked the attackers, and until the middle of the afternoon we fought around St. Suzanne. Then we got orders to by-pass this pocket of resistance and keep going toward Le Mans. It seemed strange and a little frightening to leave enemy troops behind and all around us, and to keep going deeper and deeper into the unknown.

While we were fighting around St. Suzanne that day, I remember two certain incidents. One of the British Broadcasting Company's news announcers whom we heard over one of the battalion command-post radios said: "The latest reports say that the farthest-advanced American spearheads into France are near St. Suzanne," and that was exactly where I was.

75

The other incident was a courageous act. During the morning the supply train of our regiment's first battalion was taken under fire by a group of enemy soldiers who were lying behind a bank on a road parallel to the one taken by our men. The supply train was helpless, for it could not go forward or backward. As soon as anyone got up to try to move a truck he attracted a hail of bullets.

In answer to the supply train's urgent call for help, Lieutenant Lovett, Sergeant Jake Parton and Nick (a driver) set out in a jeep from our second battalion to go to the rescue, although they had no idea how many enemy troops there were or what they might run into. By taking some back roads these three slipped up behind the Krauts and found 25 to 30 soldiers firing at the supply train. Jake blazed away with the .50-caliber machine gun mounted on the jeep while Lieutenant Lovett opened up with a tommy gun, and in a matter of seconds all the enemy soldiers were "liquidated."

That night our whole regiment was cut off when the Germans retook the one road behind us, but in the morning it was opened again.

During these confused days many strange things happened. The Germans were thoroughly disorganized and had no idea where we were, so we were constantly running into enemy staff cars with officers riding around, supply trains, rear-echelon troops and so forth. Once we captured a German colonel and his staff who were on their way to survey a location for a future defensive position. Unknown to them, we had reached the place long before the survey party did.

At Le Mans I talked with an enemy medical officer who had been on a routine inspection tour of hospitals. He was speechless with surprise when he drove gaily into the city and found himself surrounded by American troops, who no doubt were as surprised to see him as he was to find them there.

One dark night on our way across France we pulled off the road for the night. Unknown to him, one of our infantrymen lay down to sleep beside an already sleeping German soldier who had become separated from his comrades and had lain down here for the night. When the German awoke the next morning he shook the American to arouse him and then surrendered to him.

Time and again, when we'd stop for the night, the French people in whose house we'd put the aid station would tell us that a group of enemy soldiers had slept there the night before and had left only that morning. Frequently excited Frenchmen would shout *"Boche par là!"* to us as we drove by, and would point into a near-by woods, but we had no time to bother with picking up stray Jerries. Usually the F.F.I.* would pick them up.

The next day the tanks of our first battalion caught a German column of armored cars, half-tracks, trucks and several hundred German troops driving down a road, and blasted them to bits. Every enemy vehicle was knocked out and all soldiers killed, wounded or captured. The area was quite a mess. Most of the time these days our P-47's and P-51's flew protective cover over us. We'd get a report of an enemy tank column approaching on our flank, but soon our wonderful Thunderbolts would appear and dive-bomb and strafe until there were no Kraut tanks left running. We seldom saw many enemy planes during daylight, although one day a flight of 60 ME-109's came over and gave us some trouble. At night there were always quite a few Jerry planes out for some bombing, even though the German air force had been badly mauled.

Late that night, August 8, the leading elements of our battalion entered LeMans, and the next morning we marched through it in triumph. The wild, happy, riotous welcome the people gave us made us forget a little about the bitter days in Normandy. We marched north of the city a couple of miles and stopped for two or three days while the Second French Armored Division rolled through us and continued the attack to the north.

Then we hit the road again, this time marching on foot. The 358th Infantry was motorized now and we were walking along behind. We walked about 25 miles a day north for three blistering days, while the hot sun beat down and the biting dust from the French roads burned our eyes and noses. We were following along behind the Second French Armored Division, and evidences of the

---

* French Forces of the Interior, the underground organization which aided us greatly.

battle were all along the road—burned-out German and American tanks, ruined vehicles and burned buildings.

About dusk one evening, August 13, we marched through Alençon, which had just been liberated that morning. The town was packed with American troops and equipment, all milling around in the crowded streets. We moved through town and went into the fields outside it in the pitch-darkness, for the night. We were on the high ground just north of the town.

Then it all began. The Luftwaffe came over in a sizable force to bomb Alençon, and what a show! The bombers dropped flares first, lighting up the entire area with a brilliant glare which outlined every object in sharp black and white. I felt like a trapped rat in a spotlight beam as I lay helplessly on the ground under a tiny tree and without a foxhole. Oh, what a miserable feeling! There was *nothing* to do but to hope and pray and wait.

Then the bombers started to come in for their bomb runs, flying low over where I lay. As each one droned over, I prayed that those bombs wouldn't be released until after the plane had passed by. Most of the bombs did fall in or near Alençon, down in the valley. The anti-aircraft guns filled the sky with bright bursts of fire, and now and then a brilliant flash in the sky showed where a German plane had been hit by the ack-ack. Then I'd watch in fascination as it went spinning down in flames, sometimes exploding in midair.

At last my turn came—one of the bombers released a bomb over me. I heard its high-pitched whistle as it hurtled down toward me, louder and louder. It seemed like hours as I lay there waiting for it to hit. I thought, "Well, so I'm to die, after all. I wonder what the end will be like." One has a strange, calm, detached feeling at such a time. The whistle became a scream, and I opened my mouth and braced myself for the concussion. There was a dull thud and that was all. The bomb had hit very close, but it was a dud. Oh, what a relief that was! The rest of the night was quiet, so I slept soundly.

The next day our regiment was given the task of capturing the high ground to the north and cleaning out the heavy forests covering the hills. It looked like a nasty job, fighting up steep, rugged hills and through dense woods. The Second French Armored Division was already far beyond, but that force had by-passed these hills, leaving them for us to clear. However, that morning the Krauts started to pull out, and our Thunderbolts caught them on the road and "worked them over" good. All morning our planes bombed and strafed the hapless Heinies, and that afternoon we occupied the objectives without a fight. Smashed and burning Jerry guns and vehicles littered the road through the woods, and many dead soldiers were scattered around. In some of the burning vehicles sat dead Germans, being slowly cremated. When the planes had attacked this column many of the troops had fled, and now were scattered throughout the forest in small bands. We remained there about five days, rounding up prisoners. Our battalion took about 500 prisoners and killed a few Krauts, too. It seemed strange and a little eerie to hear rifle shots and the chatter of machine guns everywhere all around us in the woods as our boys rounded up the prisoners.

After all the Germans had been picked up, the regiment was motorized and started north to rejoin the rest of the division, which was driving hard to close the Falaise Gap. We proceeded to Nonant-le-Pin, where we bivouacked as the reserve regiment. The fighting up ahead was bitter, as the Krauts battled desperately to keep the trap open. For several days we sat in reserve, and then were finally committed to reinforce a spot in our lines where the enemy was launching a savage and concerted counterattack. The regiment actually did very little fighting, but I got a good look at the Falaise Pocket—a boiling, seething, flaming cauldron of hell and death.

The remnants of the German Seventh Army had been caught in a trap in a circular valley about 20 miles in diameter, surrounded by high hills. On the northern rim sat the British and on the southern rim were the Americans, blasting to bits the disorganized enemy packed in the valley. Burning tanks and vehicles, milling troops, roaring guns, heavy clouds of smoke, hundreds of dead and wounded Germans and thousands of prisoners made this a never-to-be-forgotten scene. During this action the 90th Division took more than 13,000 prisoners in four days.

After the battle was over I drove through a part of the area. Words cannot describe the terrific death and destruction—thousands of dead horses and German soldiers, roads choked with deserted or burned wagons, trucks, tanks and half-tracks, blasted artillery guns and scenes of the greatest disorganization. It was a fearful slaughter. We drove for hours through the shambles and past the silent ranks of the dead. Much of the time our jeep had to travel across the fields, for the roads were blocked by the battered and burned vehicles.

At one spot in one of the passable roads the jeep bounced over a bump in the road, which on closer inspection was seen to be a dead German. During the great slaughter he had fallen in the road, and trucks had kept rumbling over him. Now he was ground into the dirt. The many little towns in the area were ruined. Their houses were blasted and buried by the tremendous air and artillery bombardment, and their streets were made impassable by the shattered trucks and wagons and the mangled horses of the Germans.

Several times, when the people saw the Red Cross brassard on my arm, they would ask me for medical care for some of their family. Then I would make my way into the dark, damp cellar of a smashed house where civilians had huddled in terror as the battle raged, and there I would find some badly injured persons. I would give the best aid I could and go on. The public health problem must have been enormous there a few days later, with so many dead soldiers and horses lying in the summer sun, the breakdown of communications, the lack of food and the absence of medical care.

It was difficult to comprehend just how much enemy equipment had been destroyed and captured. For mile after mile we drove past guns, tanks, trucks, communication wire, tools, ammunition, office supplies, food, rolling kitchens, machine shops, clothing and so on. Many horses were running around loose, having broken from the harnesses of the German horse-drawn equipment. The scenes of chaos and wreckage were truly beyond adequate description.

I think this can be told better by quoting part of a report by Lieutenant William Mathiews, one of the 344th Field Artillery Battalion's air observers who directed fire on the enemy from a cub plane.

"On the morning of the 19th I took off to register the battalion. Just as I cleared the hills looking into the valley, I saw the roads alive with vehicles of every description. Immediately fire was brought down on the road crossing just to the north of St. Eugènie and the progress of the vehicles was stopped in that vicinity. Fire was falling in several places in the valley. However, several trucks pulled to the sides of the road and moved around the stalled vehicles, then headed north toward Chambois and St. Lambert-sur-Dives, which were under fire at that time. Every place where there were more than four vehicles grouped, artillery fire would drop. Those trucks that were still trying to escape through Chambois were piling up, caught by our fire.

"The road east of Bailleuil was blocked and the trapped vehicles began to move into the fields. The roads through Tournai-sur-Dives were blocked also, and then the roads were forgotten. Vehicles flooded out into the fields and it looked like a stampede of cattle.

"A large body of vehicles, trucks, tanks, S.P. guns, grouped south of Tournai, numbering around 200 or more. It looked as if they wanted to give up, but then they started firing, and I called for artillery. After what seemed like hours, but was actually minutes, the group of vehicles turned into Tournai. The roads were blocked and they assembled in the woods just south of town. Artillery hammered the woods until the assembly area was a mass of burning vehicles. Black smoke obscured our vision and prevented further fire at this point. The enemy gathered his vehicles along hedgerows, under trees, or out in the open. No cover was too small, but it still was not enough. Continued pressure from the rear forced them to try and move.

"Moving out into the open, and in regular lines, were several regiments of horse-drawn artillery, carts and wagons. They came forward and our first rounds landed right on them. The line wavered north of the fire and continued on. Several volleys landed right in the column and the line turned at right angles and headed north. It was a slaughter. Horses would fall and stop a wagon. Many were running away, some would turn right into the fire, others gathered in the shelter of an old rock quarry to escape but immediately artillery fire drove them out. They turned south into a crossroad just southeast of Tournai-sur-Dives and the road was soon blocked by fire. More units piled up on top of them and soon it was impossible to turn the horses. Then it became a shambles. Horses

loose and running everywhere. Some teams still hitched to cais-
sons and wagons and one or more killed in the traces. All semblance of organization had ceased at this point.

"Vehicles were still headed northeast towards the once formed
outlet of the creek but none could be seen making their way past
it. Very late in the day, another column of trucks and vehicles
tried to make Tournai-sur-Dives. They were already blocked and
turned south into other stopped vehicles. Breaks were in the column as they tried to dodge the fire, but soon they came to a halt,
and as it grew dark only occasional movement could be seen.
Grouped vehicles in Villedieu-les-Balleuil were given as interdic-
tion for the night."

One thing which surprised me was the great amount of horse-
drawn equipment the Germans had. To be sure, they had many
trucks, tanks and so forth, but the majority of their vehicles were
horse-drawn. I had heard of the German army as being such a great
mechanized juggernaut, but this was not the case. Most of their
artillery pieces and supply trains were pulled by teams of horses,
and much of their "motorized" infantry consisted of soldiers
mounted on bicycles. As a result, our completely mechanized army
was infinitely more mobile than theirs, a fact which has not been
brought out by many commentators on World War II.

For the next few days we took it easy. The Germans had collapsed in front of us, and our armored divisions were racing across
France, so we rested awhile and let them do the fighting. Then we
packed up again, left early one morning and drove 170 miles in one
day to a forest just outside Fontainebleau. It was quite a trip—a
beautiful summer day, good paved roads and crowds of cheering,
waving, flower-throwing French lining the way. When we arrived
at our destination we threw our blankets on the ground under the
huge old trees for the night's stay.

The next morning we drove through Fontainebleau (receiving a
great ovation from the populace), crossed the Seine River on pontoon bridges and continued on to Château-Thierry. The next day
we marched 20 miles north (in a pouring rain—getting soaked, of
course) and crossed the Marne River. About dark we loaded onto
trucks and rode until about 0100. Oh, how wet and cold and

miserable that long, dark ride was! About 2300 hours we drove past a burning ammunition truck, which was some little distance away. I don't know whether it was German or American, or how it was set afire, but it was quite a sight. Bursting shells lit the night sky and shook the earth with their thunder.

We finally stopped in a little town northwest of Reims. There we stayed for a couple of days and then we marched through Reims (to the cheers of the delirious natives) to another village 5 miles east of the city. We remained there for a few days, until the division was able to get enough gasoline up to us. At this point the entire Third Army had outrun its supply line and was out of gasoline.

All across France we were hailed as liberating heroes. Throngs of cheering civilians lined city streets and country roads, waving French, American and British flags, throwing flowers and kisses, pouring out wine and cider and simply going mad with joy. As we came along the F.F.I. (French Forces of the Interior), the underground, rose up to help us. Carrying captured German rifles and wearing "F.F.I." armbands, they rounded up any stray enemy soldiers and were quite a help to us. They were tough and determined, and they knew the terrain perfectly.

After a few days we loaded our vehicles with gasoline again and started east on September 5. We drove in a pouring rain into the Argonne Forest, where American troops had captured a German ammunition dump of nearly 1,000,000 tons. We remained there a day or two to guard the dump until service troops could take it over. Then we drove to and through Verdun and stopped for a wet, cold night in a small woods east of Etain. In the morning we started out again in the rain, this time on foot toward Briey. The 7th Armored Division had raced through there several days before, but after they had passed by, a large number of Krauts straggled back and got set to defend the city. Our second battalion was given the mission of taking Briey, which we did after a sharp battle for a day and a half. We hit the town early one afternoon, and found it very well defended. That night, to our north and rear, we heard a lot of tanks moving around and quite a bit of firing from tanks. Later, we learned that part of a panzer brigade had hit the division artillery command post, but had been beaten after a wild pitched battle in the dark. I heard it had hit "Divarty" pretty hard.

The next day near dark, after we had surrounded Briey, the Heinies surrendered, and we took about 500 prisoners. I entered the town with the first of our troops and visited the two hospitals, where I was greeted with wild cheers, since I was the first American soldier the patients had seen since the Krauts had come back. In one of the hospitals I found 17 wounded German soldiers—16 enlisted men and a captain. I arranged for their evacuation and sent them to the rear in a couple of trucks.

The next day we rested, and a day later we started out again on foot toward the Moselle River. The 358th Infantry headed for Thionville; we moved along abreast of them on their right, and the 359th Infantry was motorized and rushed south to back up the hard-pressed 80th Division. The 80th had established a bridgehead with two battalions across the Moselle south of Metz. Under vicious counterattacks one battalion had been pushed back into the river, but the other battalion hung onto its bridgehead with grim determination, at terrific cost. For days they fought against great odds, but they held firm. Gradually the bridgehead was expanded and made secure, but oh, the cost in American lives!

Meanwhile we moved on up to the Moselle River. The first battalion had a sharp battle around the little town of Algrange, but we hit only sporadic resistance, while the 358th entered that part of Thionville on the west bank of the river. Now, however, the Third Army was stalled before Metz. It was the sad truth that although the Krauts had abandoned Metz in the face of our onrushing columns, they had reëntered the city and its magnificent forts when we had to stop west of the city for 3 days.

We were pulled out from our position south of Thionville and thrown into futile and suicidal attacks on the great forts of Metz. Bitterly we cursed the Germans and our luck as we shivered in the fall rains, and slipped and slid in the ankle-deep mud. The poor infantrymen lying out there, soaking wet, covered with mud and under murderous fire from the forts, were really taking it again. Slowly it began to dawn on us that our sweep across France had not beaten the Krauts, and that maybe we'd have a winter war on our hands. The Allied air-borne effort in Holland had ended disastrously, and we couldn't crack Metz. We tried not to think of having to live through a winter of this hell, but we were beginning to see the bitter truth.

The second battalion was ordered to try a predawn attack. All we had to do was to cross a mile-wide, muddy, soaked field swept by machine-gun and artillery fire, traverse a deep moat filled with barbed wire, scale the walls on the other side and then assault a series of huge concrete fortresses built into a hill. It would have been suicide, so we were all greatly relieved when the attack was called off a few hours before it was to have taken place.

The rain and the mud were terrible—simply beyond description. They hampered our efforts considerably and added to our misery. After a few more days we were again moved, and took up defensive positions on the west bank of the Moselle, south of Thionville. Our battalion command post and aid station were in Amneville, which was frequently shelled by the enemy. The aid station was in an old public hall. One day during the shelling, while we were working on some wounded, a 150-mm. shell blew to bits a large concrete back porch on our building. Had the shell been a few feet higher it would have come through the wall, and no doubt killed us all. We sat there for about 3 weeks, doing little, but being shelled about twice a day. The roof of our one-story building would have given little protection against a direct hit, but luckily that never happened there.

While we were in Amneville I took care of quite a few ill and injured civilians, many of whom had been hurt by the persistent German shelling of the town. Some of the wounds were bad ones, such as was the case with the recent bride whose left arm had been shattered by the near-by explosion of a shell. I saw one 20-year-old lad who had a stiff knee as the result of an intentional injury. About a year earlier he had been ordered to report for duty with the German army, and to keep him from such forced service a physician had injected some irritant fluid (I thought the patient said gasoline) into a knee. Of course the consequence was a stiff knee. One of the boy's brothers had been taken by the Germans for military service. He had been part of an airfield defense unit in

Luxembourg, but one night, after a bombing of the field, he had slipped away and returned home to Amneville.

We were now in Lorraine which, with Alsace, had been tossed back and forth between France and Germany over the last several generations. Some of the inhabitants there had strong German leanings, although most such sympathizers had fled into the Reich upon our approach. Hitler claimed that Alsace and Lorraine really were parts of Germany, and thus, when he took them over, he decreed that only German could be spoken there and he changed the names of all the towns and of all the streets in the towns from French to German. "Adolf Hitler Platz," "Herman Göring Strasse," "Horst Wessel Strasse" and so on were to be found in every village. Lorraine of course is an industrial center, and so we saw scores of coal mines, steel mills and other factories. Göring frequently had traveled around this territory, exhorting the workers to produce more goods for *unser Führer*. In one city I visited a mansion owned by Joachim von Ribbentrop, the former champagne and wine salesman who became Germany's top Nazi diplomat.

It was on October 2, while we were in Amneville, that I was transferred from the infantry to the field artillery. I went to the 344th Field Artillery Battalion of the 90th Division, which had 105-mm. howitzers and was the supporting artillery for the 358th Infantry. I was sent there on detached service and expected to be there only a few days and then return to the infantry; but when the medical officer of that battalion did not return, I was permanently assigned to the artillery. I freely admit that I was glad of the change. Although the field artillery was no bed of roses, it was much better and safer than the infantry. When I joined the battalion it was near the village of Vionville, and had the command post and aid station in an old house. For a month we stayed there, firing on the forts around Metz.

It was while we were there that I was notified that I was to be decorated with the Silver Star for my "sortie" after the three wounded men near Portbail in Normandy in June. On the day appointed I appeared at division headquarters, with 10 or 15 other men who also were being decorated. As each man's name was read he stepped out of ranks and marched briskly to a place in front of

Major General James van Fleet, the division commander. The adjutant then read the citation, after which the general pinned the medal on the recipient, shook his hand and saluted. A cold, raw wind whipped our faces as we stood stiffly at attention, and a few raindrops spattered down from a cloud-flecked sky. In the distance we heard the roar of our artillery. As I stood there the heartbreaking, bloody misery of Normandy seemed far away, but I knew that a long, hard, cold winter lay ahead, and that in front of us the going would be as hard as anything we had faced thus far.

While we were in the Vionville area the infantry regiment (358th), which the 344th Field Artillery supported, did no attacking, but my old regiment (357th) attacked and took Mézières-les-Metz, north of Metz, after a long, vicious, bloody battle. The fight began with an attack upon a commanding slag pile, heavily defended by the Krauts. The first battalion took it in a wild charge in true western style. A brave sergeant led the attack. With a blazing pistol in each hand, he climbed up the fortified slag pile with his men close behind. Just as he reached the top, he fell dead with a bullet through his head. So it usually was with good infantrymen—if they were good soldiers they usually were killed.

After the slag pile had been taken the rest of the regiment attacked Mézières. The Germans defended it bitterly, and our advance was slow and costly. Finally, 240-mm. howitzers were brought up to fire on the town. The fire of these guns ranged methodically through town, house by house, and destroyed Mézières. I went through the town after the fight ended, and I saw that it was in complete ruins, from one end to the other. It was a nasty fight, but street fighting is always nasty.

To the south the 5th Infantry Division launched a terrific assault on Fort Driant, one of the strongest of the Metz forts. The brave men of the 5th rose to superhuman heights and fought up to the fort, but appalling losses ended their efforts in disaster. Metz still held out defiantly.

While we were in this static position before Metz, the Germans brought a huge railway gun into the city to fire at our corps headquarters many miles away. The shells passed over us on the way to the target, and they made considerable noise as they went. This was a nuisance to the corps headquarters, and the corps command was anxious to neutralize the the gun. By study of shell fragments picked up, it was possible to determine just what type of gun it was, and they then knew how much space would be required to set the gun up. A French railway man who had worked in Metz said there was only one place in the city where such a large railway gun could be set up and fired. This spot was pinpointed on the maps, and a T.O.T.* by all American guns within range was put on it. This caught the Krauts by surprise, killing part of the crew and destroying the gun.

A similar railway gun was used farther south to shell the headquarters of the Third Army. The enemy hid it in a tunnel during the day and took it out at night to fire it. However, it was neutralized by P-47 Thunderbolts which "skip-bombed" each end of the tunnel, blasting it shut and sealing the gun inside.

---

* Time-on-target, the term for a type of devastating artillery barrage. All the battalions of infantry which were to fire on the selected target were told at what second their shells were to fall on the target. They then calculated the time of flight, and fired their guns at the proper instant. As a result, a tremendous number of shells would suddenly land without warning at the same time on the hapless Germans. Occasionally, as many as 200 guns (16 or 17 battalions of artillery), ranging in caliber from 105 to 240 mm., would participate in a T.O.T. These were used very frequently, with great effect.

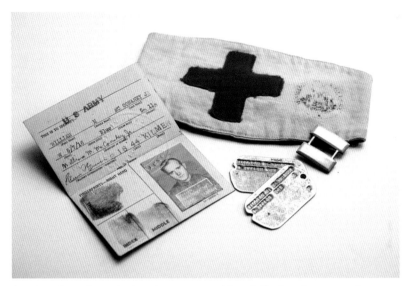

Artifacts from the author's military service: (from left) identification card, armband, captain's bars, dog tags. Courtesy of the family of William M. McConahey, M.D.

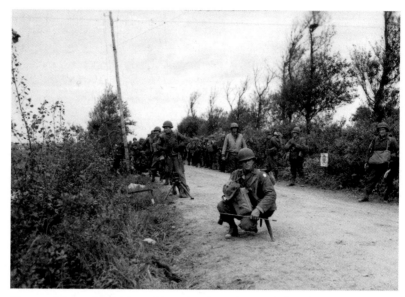

Troops of the 90th Division taking a break on the march from Utah Beach to the battle area. Note German sign denoting mine field on the right.

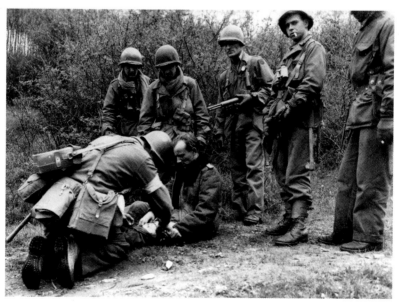

Medic treating a captured wounded German solider. Both photographs by the U.S. Army Signal Corps.

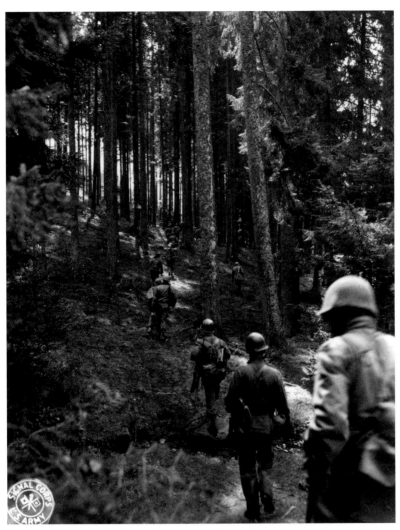

Troops of the 90th Division advancing through a woodland. Photograph by the U.S. Army Signal Corps.

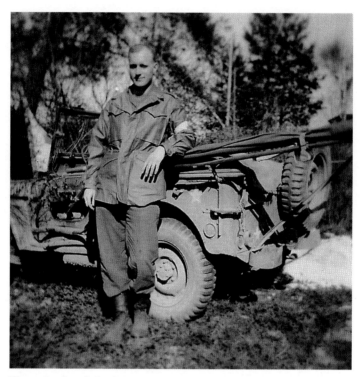

The author beside his litter jeep.

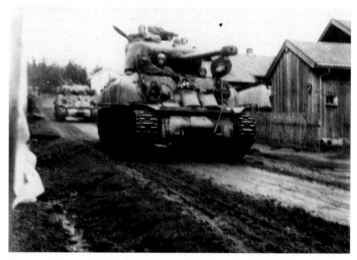

Tanks of the 712th Tank Battalion, the 90th Division's supporting armor.

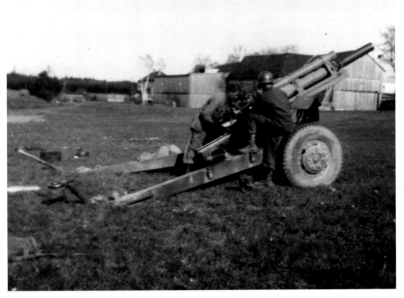

105-mm. howitzers of the 344th Field Artillery Battalion in action.

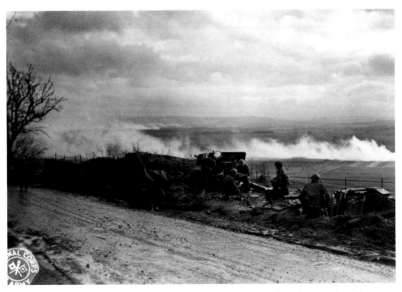

Gun of the 90th Division Tank Destroyer Battalion in place during the advance across the Saar River (hidden by smoke screen in the background) in December 1944.

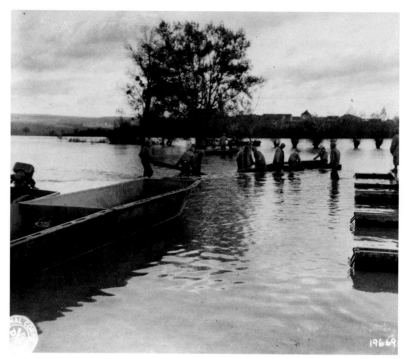
Engineers attempting to bridge the flooding Moselle River at the November 1944 crossing.

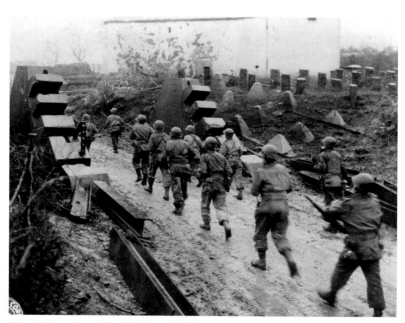
Huge "dragon's teeth" of the Siegfried Line near Habscheid, Germany. Photographs by the U.S. Army Signal Corps.

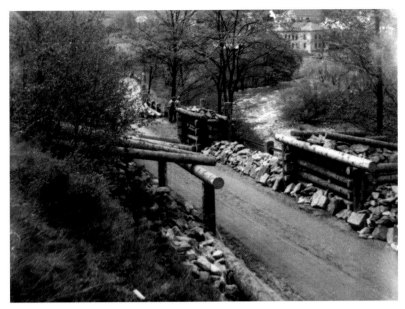

Roadblocks were prepared by the Germans against advancing forces all across Germany, but were almost never manned.

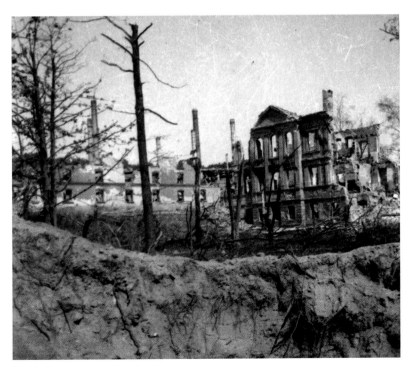

Bomb damage typical of that in most German towns in 1945.

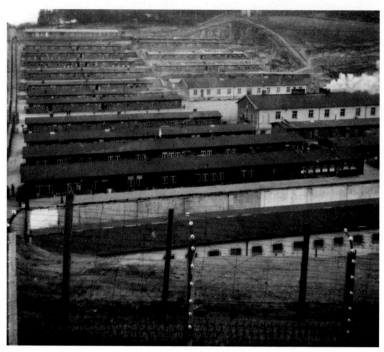

The infamous Flossenbürg Concentration Camp in April 1945.

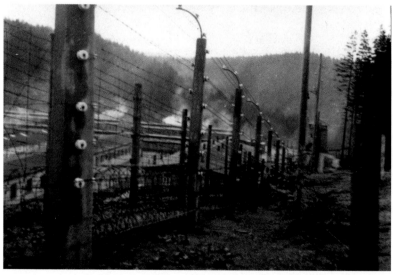

Another view of the Flossenbürg concentration camp.

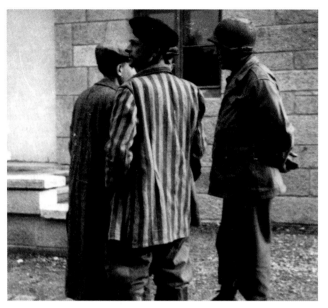

Corporal Peter Wedl, talking with inmates rescued from the
Flossenbürg Concentration Camp. Note the striped prison garb.

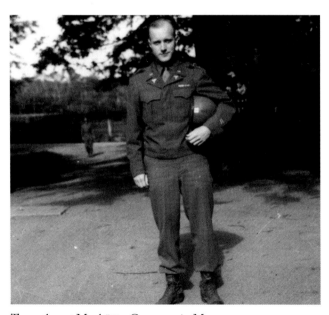

The author at Maxhütte, Germany, in May 1945.

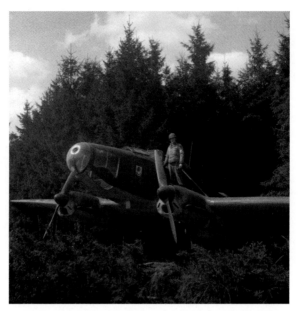

Enemy bomber at an airfield overrun by the 90th Division in April 1945.

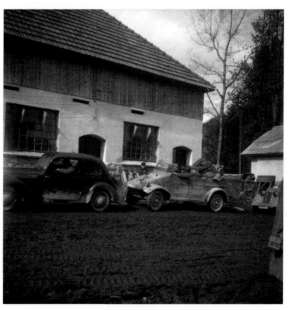

Elements of the German 11th Armored Division surrendering to the 90th Division in April 1945.

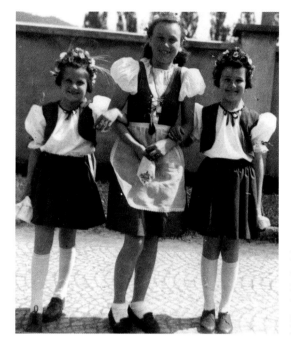

Native Czechoslovakian costumes, long forbidden by the Germans, appeared in great numbers after the liberation.

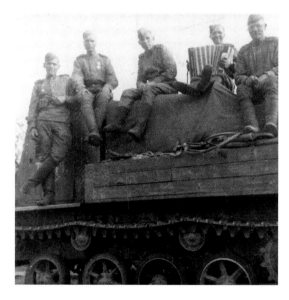

Russian troops contacted by men of the 90th Division in western Czechoslovakia in May 1945, at the meeting of the two armies.

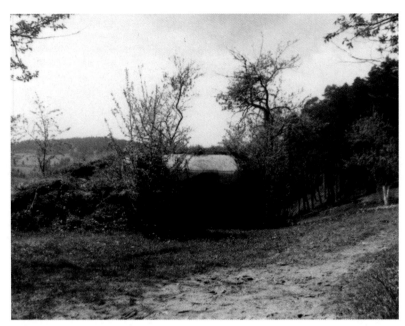

Pillbox in the Czech "Little Maginot Line" in the Sudetenland of Czechoslovakia.

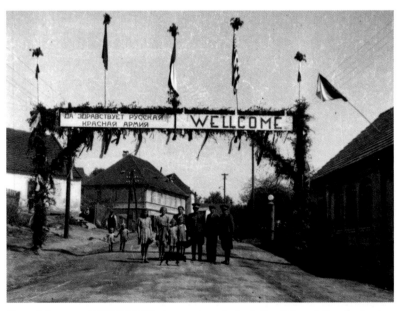

One of the many WELCOME signs written in both English and Russian in the villages of Czechoslovakia.

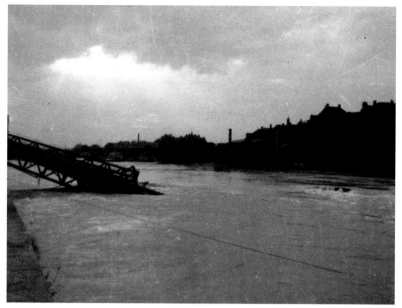

Bridges across the Danube River destroyed by retreating S.S. troops a few days before the end of the war.

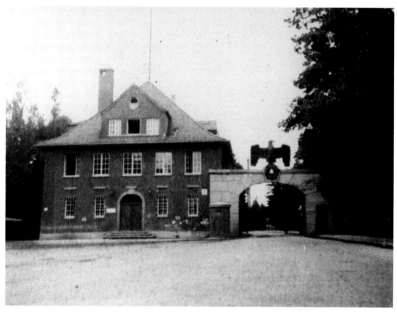

One of the entrances to the infamous Dachau Concentration Camp.

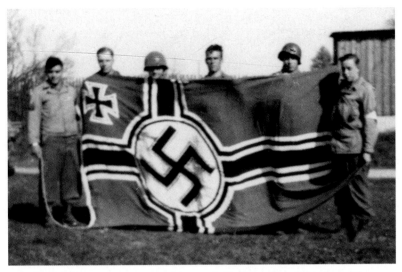

Men of the medical detachment of the 344th Field Artillery Battalion with a captured Nazi flag.

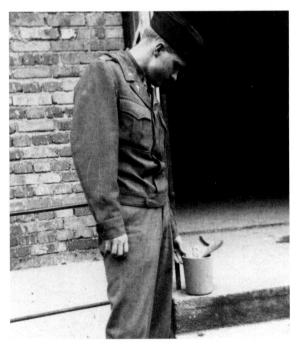

Urn containing human bones at the crematory of the Dachau Concentration Camp.

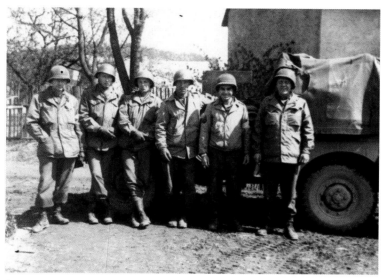

Some of the men of the medical detachment of the 344th Field Artillery
Battalion (Frazior, Mills, Jarisch, Clarin, Fortune and Wedl).

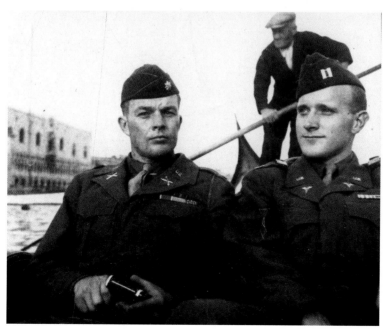

Major Swatosh and the author on the Grand Canal of Venice on a trip after
the war in September 1945.

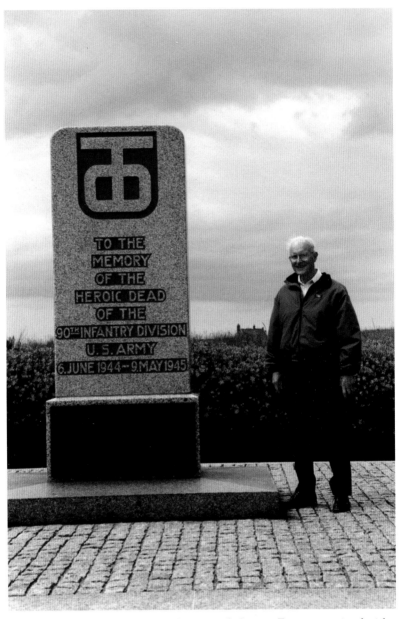

In 1999, the author and family members visited places in Europe associated with his service in World War II. This monument honors the 90th Infantry Division at its landing site on Utah Beach in Normandy, France. The insignia "TO" refers to the division's nickname, "Tough Ombres." The monument is made with granite from the Flossenbürg concentration camp, which the author helped liberate. Courtesy of the family of William M. McConahey, M.D.

Chapter Nine

THE BATTLE FOR METZ AND LORRAINE

*E*ARLY IN NOVEMBER THE 90TH DIVISION WAS replaced by the 10th Armored Division (just fresh from the States) and was pulled back for a 2 or 3 days' rest. When that happened we knew that General Patton had another tough job for us, and we weren't kept waiting long. The 20th Corps was to take Metz by swinging two circles around the city. The 90th Division was to force a bridgehead across the Moselle north of Thionville at Cattenom and link up with the 6th Armored coming up from the 80th Division's bridgehead to the south, while the 95th and 5th Infantry Divisions were to swing a tight circle around Metz and enter the city.

Several days before the attack was to begin, General Patton visited all the divisions which were to participate. Some of the officers of the 90th were assembled to hear "Georgie's" pep talk, which went something like this: "I've been going up and down the line today giving hell to everybody, but I don't need to chew out you bastards. I just stopped by to say hello, because I thought you'd be insulted if I didn't. There's nothing I can tell you sons-of-bitches. You bastards sure know how to fight! You always do more than I ask you to, and I ask plenty! You have a damn good fighting outfit. Just keep on doing as you have been and you'll be all right."

Patton was proud of the 90th Division, and frequently said so publicly. At a 3rd Army meeting of all corps and division commanders during the Battle of the Bulge he said that his best infantry division was the 90th and that his best armored division was the 4th Armored. Patton was strictly a "front-line" general. Time and again I saw him riding around up front in his jeep, with the three stars on the bright red background gleaming on the front bumper. We 3rd Army men swore by "Georgie," and had complete confidence in his great leadership.

The 90th Division was to cross the Moselle November 9, so several days before that, the division moved secretly at night to the point of attack near Cattenom and got "under cover." All the division symbols on our helmets and uniforms were covered, as were the "90's" on the vehicles. Our artillery battalion's command post and aid station were in one of the large underground forts of the Maginot Line, and there I lived for about 10 days. It was quite an interesting place, with its moats, steel doors, disappearing machine-gun turrets, gun ports, thick concrete walls, deep subterranean rooms and so forth.

The weather as usual was terrible—cold, muddy and pouring rains. The mud was worst of all. I knew how the infantry would be feeling. The miserable weather and the nasty job ahead would not make their lot any easier. Then, too, there is always such a feeling of loneliness in the infantry. There seem to be so few of you in any one place. The farther to the rear you go, the more people and activity you see—artillery battalions, bustling supply trains, rushing messengers, rear-echelon troops; but up there at the front you don't see many people. There is a strange, disquieting feeling of being alone—alone with the enemy and with death.

Before daylight the morning of November 9 the attack began. Our infantry crossed the river in rubber assault boats (in a cold, drizzling rain) without previous artillery preparation, catching the Germans by surprise. By daylight our boys had a good toehold on the east bank, and by nightfall all three infantry regiments were across.

But then nature hit us a crack. Because of the heavy rains the Moselle River began to rise and within a few hours we had the worst Moselle flood in 50 years. When the first infantrymen slipped across the river before dawn it was a swift-flowing stream a couple of hundred yards wide, but by evening it had become a raging torrent nearly a mile across, over which the engineers were unable to put a bridge. As a result, the infantrymen were really "on their own." How those soldiers ever lasted out those next few days I'll never know, isolated as they were. They had no overcoats, raincoats or blankets to protect them from the cold and the driving rain; they had no overshoes to keep their feet dry in the deep mud; very little food or ammunition could be sent across the rampaging river; the wounded could not be brought back across the flood; no tanks or antitank guns could get over. Yet those boys stood fast against the fury of desperate counterattacks, threw back the enemy and advanced across heavily mined fields in the face of fanatical resistance.

The key to the enemy defenses in this area was Fort Königs-macher, one of the most formidable forts I've ever seen. It was a series of steel and concrete strongpoints built into the top of a commanding hill, and so well concealed that little could be seen of it above ground. Underground passages, dozens of machine-gun emplacements, antitank ditches, four disappearing 150-mm. artillery pieces and so forth made it an extremely strong fort. But it fell to the undying courage and determination of the infantry. Some of the boys of the 358th Regiment fought their way to the top of it, poured burning gasoline into the ventilators, blew open the massive steel doors with composition C and routed out the Boche. Because of the heavy casualties sustained during the advance to the fort our commanders had decided to call off the attack, but the infantry had refused to quit and had pushed on until the fort was theirs.

Still the raging river prevented help from getting across to the hard-pressed combat soldiers. The artillery cub planes dropped medical supplies, composition C and blankets to the troops across the river, but the planes were able to carry only a pitifully small amount. At last, however, the river began to recede, and the engineers started to work on two bridges: one in our area at Cattenom and one down the river several miles where the 359th Infantry had crossed.

Shortly before the bridge down the river was completed the Jerries launched a smashing counterattack against the 359th, using tanks and infantry, aimed at splitting our bridgehead and blowing up the bridge across the river. It was a violent attack which nearly succeeded. We still had no antitank guns across, and the infantry-men couldn't stop the onslaught with bazookas. Enemy tanks overran the infantry, shooting the boys pointblank in their fox-holes. The fire of every available artillery piece was turned on this counterattack until 17 battalions of our artillery were blasting the advancing enemy. Germans dropped like flies and tank after tank was disabled under the murderous artillery fire, but still they came on. Finally the counterattack was broken and the enemy was routed. A few German soldiers straggled back, but most of the attackers lay dead, and their tanks were burning hulks.

The next day our bridge across the river at Cattenom was fin-ished and the 344th Field Artillery was ordered to cross it that night. Shortly after midnight we started down the road toward the bridge. It was a cold, windy night alternating between rain and snow. Of course it was pitch-black except when the sky was lighted by stabbing flashes from the big guns of both sides. It was a long, slow trip, for in the darkness vehicles frequently slipped off the muddy roads into deep ditches, delaying traffic until they were pulled out at the cost of much labor and a number of colorful expletives.

Just about the time my jeep had almost reached the bridge a gun truck got stuck, and so for about an hour we sat there, packed bum-per to bumper, while the truck was being worked on. During this delay the Jerries dropped in a battery volley (four shells), trying to hit the bridge, but they were short. It was rather nerveracking to sit there helplessly in the darkness, packed in like sardines, and wait. Yet there was nothing else to do. At last our column started again and my jeep got on the pontoon bridge. It was a long bridge and the roaring river gurgled angrily around the pontoons, but we got across safely.

Soon after we got over, the truck ahead of us stopped. I found that the driver had lost the convoy in the darkness. None of us knew which road to take, nor did we know where the enemy was, except that he was rather close. We did know that the entire area was heavily mined. Finally we started out on the road which seemed to me to be the correct one, and after several tense minutes we found the rest of the battalion. The guns were pulling off the road into position and I took my medical section into an old house and set up an aid station in a room across the hall from the command post.

Now the infantry pushed ahead fast, and we moved frequently in order to give them close support. The Germans still fought bitterly and launched many small but fierce counterattacks. One of these recaptured a town for a short time, but our boys soon took the village back. I entered the town soon afterward and saw that the Heinies had paid heavily for their futile efforts. German dead littered the streets, and outside the town scores of German soldiers lay dead in the fields where our accurate artillery fire had caught them in the open. So thick were the dead that when I walked across the field I had trouble walking around or stepping over the bodies. Some of course were horribly mutilated. Apparently this group of soldiers had been caught by our artillery just as they were starting to dig foxholes. They never had a chance.

In a dark shed on a dilapidated farm about a mile outside of town I found two badly wounded Kraut soldiers lying on piles of potatoes. I gave them first aid and sent them back to the rear. Of course the town had been badly damaged, as had all towns through there, where the fighting was so heavy.

Two days later we made contact with the 6th Armored Division. The 5th and 95th divisions had entered Metz and the battle for that fortress was over. For the first time in history Metz had fallen to an attacking force.

While the rest of the division swung directly east and continued the advance, our combat team (358th Infantry and 344th Field Artillery) were sent north to help the 10th Armored Division. They had crossed the Moselle behind us, pushed north up the "triangle" between the Saar and Moselle rivers and crossed the border into Germany. But they had not gone far. Just north of Borg they had been stopped by the Siegfried Line.

We set up headquarters in the town of Perl, Germany, and for the next week our infantry fought a series of weird, bloody battles in this part of the Siegfried Line. We were to open a way through the "dragon's teeth" and pillboxes for the tanks of the 10th Armored. It was tough going for our tired, depleted battalions, whose rifle companies were at about half-strength, not yet having received replacements for the casualties around Metz. In spite of the difficulties the boys did well and made good progress, although the cost in lives was heavy. As usual, many unsung heroes in the infantry did their jobs well and died so that we could advance—such as the remaining members of a company who were cut off in a little town. Even though they were facing disaster they refused to surrender and fought from cellar to cellar while enemy tanks blew down the houses above them. Although our boys did open the way, the 10th Armored failed to follow through, so that our efforts and our heavy casualties there were in vain. After this fiasco we rejoined the rest of the division back across the border in France, pushing rapidly toward the Saar River.

While we were in Perl I saw a small prison camp which had housed American prisoners of war. It was empty now, but the barbed-wire fences, dilapidated barracks and empty cardboard American Red Cross P.O.W. boxes told the grim story. I wondered who the lads were who had been there and where they were now.

It was about this time that a large flight of B-26's came over us fairly low, to bomb around the German town of Merzig on the Saar. One of the bombers was hit by flak and we watched it as it slowly circled earthward with smoke trailing from it. All the crew jumped to safety and all landed behind American lines. We watched the airmen float to earth in their parachutes and our battalion picked up a couple of them. One of these was the pilot, with whom I talked.

During these winter days we often saw V-2 weapons (the rocket bombs) being launched many miles to the east. We could not see the rockets themselves, but we saw the long trails of white smoke as the weapons mounted higher and higher in the sky and headed toward installations in our rear. Earlier in France we frequently had seen the V-1's (the buzz bombs) "put-putting" overhead. These weapons never were used on the front-line troops, however. They were always aimed toward the rear.

Early in December we entered Germany again and closed up to the Saar, but we did not pause there long. The division was ordered to cross the river and take Dillingen in one of the strongest and widest parts of the Siegfried Line, at a place where the Siegfried Line came right down to the edge of the river. On the dark night of December 6 the infantry crossed the river in assault boats and stormed ashore. How they did it in the face of myriads of cross-firing pillboxes I don't know, but they knocked out many pillboxes and by dawn were well entrenched. After daylight the troops were harrassed by pillboxes in their rear that had been bypassed in the first rush to get as far inland as possible, but gradually these were reduced.

Then followed two weeks of bitter fighting in miserable winter weather. Slowly the Americans inched forward, knocking out scores of pillboxes and taking most of Dillingen. It was a herculean task, achieved at great cost to us.* Because of the heavy enemy artillery fire no bridge could be thrown across, and so ferries were built to carry across T.D.'s† and supplies. They operated shrouded in a continuous smoke screen. Slowly, however, the Siegfried Line was cracking.

Then came December 17 and the bad news. Hourly the reports came in about the great Ardennes counteroffensive, and the picture became blacker and blacker. If the Krauts kept on coming and cut down behind the 3rd Army we'd be in a bad spot. The 90th Division, with all three regiments across the Saar and engaged in the Siegfried Line, had little with which to protect its rear. On December 19 came the order to give up all our hard-won gains and pull back across the river. The infantrymen hated this order because retreat was not to their liking, especially when they were winning.

---

* Dillingen itself was a fortress, studded with many camouflaged pillboxes. An innocent-appearing jewelry store, a hardware store, a railway ticket office and many other such buildings scattered through town turned out to be steel and concrete pillboxes.
† Tank destroyers, which were heavy guns mounted on half-track or full-track vehicles.

Yet the withdrawal of the division was a masterpiece. It is a most difficult maneuver to disengage a division and withdraw without sustaining heavy casualties, but the 90th got back across the Saar without any trouble and before the Heinies realized what was going on. We moved at once to hold part of the defense line facing north between the Saar and the Moselle rivers. Our G-2 reports indicated that possibly the Germans might launch another counterattack from the area behind the Siegfried Line between the Saar and the Moselle against the 3rd Army, and we were there to stop it.

The next two weeks were ones of anxious watching and waiting, although we did little work. The Ardennes counteroffensive to the north kept on rolling and the weather remained cloudy, grounding our air force. We prepared a strong defense in our sector—mined the fields, wired bridges and roads for demolition, prepared trees to be blown down for roadblocks, selected alternate positions to be used if we had to retreat and posted numerous road guards.

In the area of the 1st Army, jeeploads of English-speaking German soldiers in American uniforms roamed around in the rear of the lines spreading confusion, killing officers and destroying army installations. Hence, in our area many check points were set up on the roads to prevent such aggressions from happening to us. We were alerted for anything—paratroop landings, secret agents behind our backs, an attack by panzer divisions—but all was quiet on our front. We spent Christmas and New Year's there. In the meantime it had become very cold and we had lots of snow and ice. Then the clouds broke and we had a long stretch of clear weather, during which our air force pounded the Germans in the "Bulge" unceasingly.

While we were in that location I had the first shower bath I had had for many months. About 10 miles to the rear a quartermaster detachment had set up a shower-bath unit which all the men in our battalion were permitted to visit, a few at a time. Three of my men and I drove back for baths one bitterly cold day. The temperature was below zero, so we were none too warm as we stripped off our clothes in the "undressing" tent, even though there was a coal stove in the center. Then we ran into the shower tent, where hot water sprayed from multiple holes in several long pipes. It felt wonderful to scrub up again, but it was a different feeling when we ran back to the dressing tent to dry off and get dressed in the freezing air. However, I didn't have to worry much about baths. My next shower was not to come for another two or three months.

It was remarkable that we kept so free from lice. The reason was DDT powder. Every man had a can of DDT powder with which to dust himself once a week, and this controlled the lice to a great extent. Of course, now and then men would become mildly infested. I had lice twice myself, but prompt application of additional powder eliminated the pests in short order. Scabies appeared constantly among our men, with great frequency, but luckily this parasite missed me.

Chapter Ten

THE BATTLE OF THE BULGE

ALL ALONG WE HAD KNOWN THAT SOONER OR later the old 90th would be sent up to the Ardennes battle where the fighting was so bitter and so difficult, and soon we got our orders. We were to move secretly and attack the enemy by surprise. The 94th Division came in to relieve us, so we covered our division symbols and "90's" and quickly started north on January 7. We drove more than 100 miles that day in heavy snow and terrible cold, during which drive I got so cold in my open jeep that I thought I'd freeze. I did get my toes and fingers frostbitten sometimes during the Ardennes campaign. Every time I rode in my jeep during the entire winter my feet became numb with cold, for I literally rode with my feet on a cake of ice. The sandbags which had been put on the floor of the jeep for protection in case we hit a mine became thoroughly soaked in the fall rains. When the weather turned cold the soggy bags froze solidly and remained frozen until spring came. Thus my feet rested upon a block of ice whenever I rode in a jeep.

We drove from Gongelfangen to Waldmünchen to Cattenom to Luxembourg City and then to a little town in Luxembourg a few miles northeast of Bastogne, Belgium. We moved into position between the 6th Armored Division on our left and the 26th Infantry Division on our right, and got set for a surprise attack at dawn on January 9. For many days the 26th had been battering against crack enemy troops on this southern flank of the salient without progress. They assured us that the 90th would be lucky to advance 100 yards.

At dawn our boys jumped off, and by dark they had driven the Germans back 2½ miles. We caught them by surprise, for so successful had been our secret move that the enemy did not know that a fresh division had come into the line. The next 6 weeks were as miserable as any we ever lived through. The bitter cold, the deep snow, the howling blizzards, the mountainous terrain we were fighting across and the bloody, bitter fighting made it a hell we'll never forget. Although I was uncomfortable, my discomfort was insignificant when compared to that of our infantry. I wondered how those boys ever stood it at all—night after night in cramped, icy foxholes, weeks of ferocious attack and counterattack, only cold K rations to eat, and all the rest. Words can't describe the miseries those boys suffered. Trench foot and frozen limbs hospitalized many, and some wounded men froze to death before they could be rescued.

Even so, our boys pressed steadily onward, sometimes advancing across frozen, snow-covered fields which had been turned black by the explosions of hundreds of enemy shells. The Germans fought skilfully and hard to hold their gains in the wild, snowy mountains of the Ardennes. One titanic battle I still remember. Our artillery battalion was in position around Bras, Belgium. The infantry was a couple of miles ahead of us, having just taken the Luxembourg towns of Niederwampach and Oberwampach, key points in the German defense system. The Krauts were ordered to retake Oberwampach at any cost, so during the night they threw all available S.S. troops into a violent counterattack. For 24 hours the battle flamed and swirled in the cold and snow in and around the town. Wave after wave of screaming, fanatical enemy soldiers accompanied by tanks and tank destroyers smashed at our men. Point-blank tank duels, street fighting, bayonet encounters and heavy artillery fire made Oberwampach a village of horror and sudden death; but our boys held firm and the Germans could not crack our line.

Much credit must be given to the artillery for stopping this counterattack. The guns put up a curtain of steel in front of the town, and Jerries dropped by the score as they came running across the open fields. All night and all day our guns thundered. During this 24-hour period the 344th Field Artillery Battalion fired nearly 3,500 rounds of ammunition, the most it ever fired in a 24-hour span. Bringing up ammunition to the spitting howitzers over the snow-clogged country roads was a tremendous task for the service troops, but the ammunition got to us. Later, after the infantry had moved ahead the artillery went into position around Oberwampach. The town was a shambles, and in the surrounding fields I counted more than 20 knocked-out enemy tanks. Dead German soldiers lay everywhere, many of them ugly masses of torn flesh and bone, ripped to pieces by our murderous artillery fire.

During the terrible battle in Oberwampach a brave sergeant from the 344th Field Artillery Battalion who was a member of a forward observation party with the infantry gave his life for a little Luxembourg child. He had taken refuge in the cellar of a smashed house, along with the family who owned the house. Outside, a barrage of Kraut shells crashed down. Suddenly, a terror-stricken child darted out the door into that hail of steel. Without a moment's hesitation the sergeant dashed after the child, gathered the little fellow up in his arms and started back for the safety of the cellar. Just then a 120-mm. mortar shell exploded near by. The sergeant was mortally wounded but the child was unhurt. "Greater love hath no man than this, that a man lay down his life for his friend."

It was sad to see the destruction of so many pretty little Belgian and Luxembourg towns. Many of them were battered and burned beyond recognition. There is nothing else like the desolation of a war-ruined village—the shattered, smoldering buildings, the rubble-covered streets, the dead soldiers lying here and there, the dazed civilians huddled in dark, cold, damp cellars, the battered, discarded equipment of battle strewn about, and the stench of death. It is all a gruesome nightmare that etches itself forever in one's brain. The little town of Bras, Belgium, was as completely destroyed as any village I saw. It was located on a hillside beside the main highway running east from Bastogne, and the Germans had fought madly to keep the road open, using Bras as a bulwark. Our artillery had shelled it unceasingly and our

P-47's had dive-bombed it frequently. When I moved into it to set up an aid station there was little shelter to be found. In the entire town there was only one room with four walls and a roof, all intact. The rest of the house was a crumbling ruin, but we used that one room for the aid station. All around us were heaps of wreckage—houses that had been hit directly by bombs—with arms, legs and heads of dead Germans protruding grotesquely from the débris. Directly in front of the house we used lay a dead enemy soldier on his back, his hands thrown up, his face a bloody mass and his right leg blown off at the midthigh. Other battered corpses were ground into the frozen earth. The nauseating stench was intolerable to us, and so we were glad when a heavy snow blanketed the ugly sights and colder weather decreased the odor of putrefaction somewhat.

Sometimes, when I came across recently killed German soldiers, I would look through some of the belongings scattered around on the snow near the fallen bodies. It always gave me a strange feeling to see letters from families, wives and sweethearts and to look at pictures of children and family groups. The men we fought had loved ones at home, hoping and praying for their safe return, just as we had. It seemed like a crazy world.

After the terrific counterattack at Oberwampach had failed, the Germans fell back rapidly to the northeast through Luxembourg for some miles. They fought only a delaying action back to the Siegfried Line. However, some of the "delaying actions" fought while we were closing up to the Siegfried Line were plenty tough. We moved slowly but steadily through the heavy snow to Asselborn and then Boxhorn. It was in Boxhorn that I spent another bad night. Although our infantry was a good distance out in front of us, our right flank was open, for the 26th Division on our right had not pushed ahead as fast as we had. As a result, the Krauts could throw in a lot of artillery from close range on our right. We had the aid station in the rickety town schoolhouse. About dark we climbed into our bedrolls and huddled in our blankets, trying to keep warm in the biting cold—and then it started. The Jerries tossed in some shells too close for comfort and kept it up for the rest of the night. Most of the rounds seemed to land up and down the road in front of the schoolhouse. To make things worse, the only protection we had in the school was a thin wall mostly taken up by high windows from which the glass had been smashed. A shell hitting the side of the house could have killed us all. After a couple of shells hit within 15 yards of us, sending steel fragments screaming through the gaping windows, I decided I'd better move the aid station to a more substantial location. I made a quick reconnaissance in the dark, between shells, and selected a solid stone building not far away. Then we hurriedly moved the aid-station equipment to the new location and settled down for a cold, miserable night of "sweating out" continuous shellfire.

It was a most unpleasant night, although we felt fairly safe in our stone building. I guess it's just as well we didn't find out until morning (after the shelling ceased) that a huge supply of T.N.T. was piled up beside the building in which we had taken refuge.

From Boxhorn we moved on up through Trois Vierges to the northern tip of Luxembourg, crossed a narrow neck of Belgium and once more entered Germany, closely following the retreating Krauts. It was at Burg Reuland, Belgium, that the division smashed across the Ourthe River into Germany and the Siegfried Line again.

About this time I was hit by an extremely bad attack of gastroenteritis. Severe vomiting and diarrhea and a temperature of 104 degrees made me feel very ill. After a few days I felt better, but for a while I was really knocked out.

Chapter Eleven

THROUGH THE SIEGFRIED LINE

*N*OW THE BATTLE TO SMASH THE SIEGFRIED LINE began—a fight that was against adverse weather conditions as well as against Germans. It was cold, but not quite cold enough to freeze—this February in 1945. Rain fell continually and things were in a muddy mess. Most of us were mud from head to foot, unshaven, tired and plagued by recurrent epidemic severe diarrhea. As did many of our soldiers, I had diarrhea about half the time most of the winter. It was bad enough during the day, but at night it was even more unpleasant. It was miserable to have to jump from one's blankets three or four times a night, hastily put on boots, run outside into the cold and rain and wade through the mud in the dark to the straddle pit. As likely as not the enemy would be shelling the area, and that did not help.

Epidemics of diarrhea, often accompanied by severe abdominal cramps and occasionally by vomiting and fever, swept up and down the front, sometimes seriously hampering the fighting efficiency of the army. The causation was never known, but it appeared to be an air-borne virus. Contamination of food and water could not have been the cause. We could not keep enough bismuth and paregoric in the aid station to treat the hordes of patients.

As usual, it was the infantrymen who really suffered in the nasty fighting. Cold, wetness, mud and hunger day after day; vicious attack and counterattack; sleepless nights in muddy foxholes; and the unending rain made their life a special hell. The supply problems were terrific. Mud roads simply disappeared under the heavy army traffic and rain. The engineers worked feverishly day and night throwing rocks and logs into muddy morasses, but they waged a losing battle. Soon most of the roads in our area were almost impassable and some were completely closed. In one place the rails of a railway were torn up and the bed was used as a supply road. In an effort to relieve the acute problem of supply, fleets of C-47's flew in and dropped supplies to us by parachute.

In spite of the weather, our attack continued. The 90th Division crashed into the Siegfried Line in the vicinity of Habscheid and bored slowly ahead through the "dragon's teeth," numerous pillboxes and heavy enemy fire. To our left the 4th Division took Brandscheid and then swung northeast. Our combat team relieved the 4th in Brandscheid and continued the advance east. The aid station now was in a little town about a mile from Brandscheid, but I could see that town very clearly across a valley on the next hill. It had been battered out of existence by our bombing and shelling, and now that our troops had taken it the Germans were shooting at it. I stood by my aid station, listening and watching as barrages of "screaming meemies"* howled in, blanketing the town under a curtain of high explosives and death. Gradually the fire slackened as the enemy fell back in the Siegfried Line. Soon the artillery moved forward and I set up an aid station in Habscheid. It was difficult to find an intact room in this shattered town, formerly a strong-point in the Siegfried Line, but we had to have a place inside, out of the rain, to operate an aid station. Finally we set up in one "good" room in an otherwise wrecked house. The town was a mess, as were all the towns in the area. All buildings were in ruins, débris was scattered far and wide and the unpaved streets had been made seas of mud by the steady rains.

---

* "Screaming meemies" was the nickname given the rockets fired by the *Nebelwerfers*. These German guns had six barrels arranged in a circle, from which six rockets were fired simultaneously. Since as a rule four to six guns were fired in volleys, 24 to 36 rockets were launched together. As they traveled through the air the rockets emitted a weird, frightening, high-pitched scream which became louder as they approached. The rockets had a tremendous concussion, but little fragmentation.

On our left the 4th Division smashed into Prüm and the 90th shattered the Siegfried Line in our sector, driving to the Prüm River. Then, to our dismay, we were pulled out, moved south and ordered to crack the Line again in a new area. This our great infantrymen did in record time once more. Good use was made of the self-propelled 155's, which were 155-mm. rifles mounted on half-tracks. One of these would drive up to within range of a pillbox, fire a few rounds at it and then withdraw before the Krauts could get a bead on it with their artillery. Two or three rounds from one of these giants often was enough to crack open a pillbox. Sometimes the infantry took the pillboxes unaided, using their bazookas and T.N.T. The boys got to be extremely skilled at taking the pillboxes one after another in record time. Now that we had breached the vaunted Siegfried Line the division was relieved by the 6th Armored Division and was given a six-day rest. Just before we pulled out I had a narrow escape from being blown up by a mine. I was driving down a road in my jeep with the battalion commander's reconnaissance party when we came upon two of our light tanks which had run onto Teller mines in the road and had been knocked out. We gingerly drove into a field around the tanks and back onto the road in front of them. A short time later a jeep which came along over our same path hit a mine which all of us miraculously had straddled. The man beside the driver (where I sat in my jeep) was killed. A leg was torn off and his body was hurled 300 yards by the force of the explosion.

One day toward the end of the cracking of the Siegfried Line, when we had the Germans on the run, I had a good chance to watch a full-scale battle. The infantry had been moving ahead rapidly and our artillery had gone into position close behind them. So close were we that our guns were on one hillside while across the valley on the other slope were the Jerries. I sat in the ruins of an old house on the hill watching the battle. I saw our tanks and tank destroyers firing on enemy troops, German soldiers fleeing up the hill and the shells from the guns of our battalion exploding across the valley. After dark the tracer bullets from the machine guns of both sides and the red flash of the bursting shells made a brilliant picture. We got a few Kraut shells thrown our way, but the enemy was too disorganized and doubtless too confused to be able to concentrate much artillery on us.

It was about this time that "artificial moonlight" was used for the first time. Sometimes on cloudy nights two or three powerful searchlights far in the rear would be turned on, with their beams pointed skyward. Reflected light from the overhanging clouds would give a very dim glow to the country for miles around, much like that on a moonlit night, thus allowing traffic behind the front to move much more easily and safely in the darkness and enabling the front line troops to see enemy movements in front of them.

Our six-day rest was all too short, but we enjoyed it while it lasted. We got showers, clean underwear and clean uniforms, and best of all, we had a respite from roaring guns and screaming shells. Then we were back at it again. We relieved the 6th Armored Division and continued the advance east. It was hard driving over the miserable muddy roads, and more than once we had to get off the jeep to push it out after it was mired down. However, we moved ahead faster and faster all the time, now that the Siegfried Line was behind us. There was still one more good-sized river, the Kyll, in front of us before we could start for the Rhine, and we expected the enemy to make a stand along this river. Our division moved up to it in preparation for an assault crossing. At this particular time the 358th Infantry was in reserve, so the 344th Field Artillery was supporting the 357th Infantry Regiment. We moved into a small town not far from the river and fired for the infantrymen as they advanced toward the river. We could hear the rattle of small-arms fire and the howl of the "screaming meemies" up ahead, but no shots came our way.

The next day the 358th Infantry was ordered to cross the Kyll at Gerolstein, several miles to the north. During the morning our battalion displaced north, driving along an exposed "ridge road" parallel to the river. Across the river in plain view was hill after hill of enemy territory—a perfect place from which German observers could direct devastating artillery fire on our slowly moving column. As we drove along I waited expectantly for the zip and crash of those shells, but incredibly, they never came. When we arrived at our destination I realized that the enemy must have retreated from the river, otherwise they would have blown us to bits. Soon the infantrymen started to wade across the narrow river against no opposition. Their mission was to secure a good bridge-head for the passage of the 11th Armored Division through us.

About this time we learned that the 4th Armored Division to the south had crossed the Kyll and broken loose, and was rampaging to the Rhine. This explained the sudden collapse of resistance in front of us. The next day the artillery was ordered to cross the Kyll and join the infantrymen on the other side of Gerolstein. Since the 11th Armored had started to cross the bridge the engineers had built, we had to drive several miles down the river and cross another engineer bridge. On the other side of the river the muddy road we took to Gerolstein wound up and down over steep hills and through heavy woods. It was a rainy, misty day and the whole business seemed weird and strange as we went through dark, ghostly forests and drove past many deserted German artillery trucks and much scattered equipment.

We stayed in Gerolstein for a couple of days while the 11th Armored Division passed through us. It seemed good to let the armored boys carry the ball again, and to relax and simply sit and watch the tanks roll by. One night I heard not far away one of the heaviest and longest artillery bombardments I ever heard. I couldn't tell whether it was "incoming mail" or our artillery firing on a German counterattack against the 11th Armored. The next day I learned it was the latter. The barrage was tremendous and it smashed the Kraut attack.

As soon as all the 11th Armored had gone by we started out again, this time for the Rhine River. As we drove down the road we passed thousands of bedraggled German soldiers marching to the rear. All had been disarmed, but the guards were few and far between. However, few guards were needed. The 11th Armored had cut the Krauts to pieces and the remaining enemy troops were quite willing to surrender.

On we rushed toward the Rhine, meeting almost no opposition, for the condition of the enemy troops against us was chaotic. By the time the guns of our artillery battalion were in position one place, our infantry already would have moved ahead out of range, so we'd pack up and move again—and so on and on several times each day. The weather was still cold and it rained most of the time, but we didn't mind the weather now that we had the Krauts on the run. Terror-stricken German civilians put up white flags on their houses and waved white handkerchiefs in token of surrender as we roared by. Every now and then along the roads we passed the wreckage of German army columns caught and destroyed by the guns of the racing tanks ahead of us. Smashed wagons, dead horses and enemy soldiers and battered trucks littered the roads.

Through Schonehen and Kelberg we drove, and then into the ruins that had been Mayen before our bombers came. From Mayen we drove northeast and stopped a couple of miles from the Rhine, with our guns in position to shoot across the river. While we sat there for a couple of days waiting for further orders, I decided to drive up to see the Rhine River, and so one day Peter Wedl (my driver) and I drove to near-by Andernach, which was on the west bank and had been taken by the 11th Armored. There was still some fighting and sniping going on in the town, so we stayed out of the center of the place and drove down to the river through the edge of town. We parked the jeep, walked across a couple of fields and there it was—the mighty Rhine River of song and fable. It was wide and swift-flowing, and across the water tall hills rose steeply from its banks. From a little town on the slope of the hill and from the tops of the towering cliffs Heinie snipers shot across the river and directed sporadic artillery fire on Andernach, so we didn't linger long. It wasn't worth being killed just to look at the Rhine. At the edge of town on the way out we stopped at a *Luft-waffe* hospital—a large, rambling barracks-type affair with many deep, underground, bombproof rooms. In a couple of the under-ground rooms were wounded German soldiers, but the rest of the hospital was occupied as barracks by hundreds of foreign slave laborers from all nationalities of conquered Europe.

Chapter Twelve

THE SECOND CROSSING OF THE MOSELLE

*T*HE NEXT DAY THE BATTALION MOVED TO THE little town of Münstermaifield a couple of miles from the Moselle River. We soon were given the plans for the next operation. The 90th Division was to make another assault-crossing of the Moselle at Brodenbach. The Third Army was to cross the river from west to east, south of Koblenz, and drive down into the Palatinate to link up with the Seventh Army and trap a large number of Jerries in a huge bag. Before dawn on the morning of March 14 our troops slipped across the river in assault boats and the battle was on again. We were facing the Sixth S.S. Mountain Division (called *Nord,* I think), but they were spread too thinly to do us great harm, and the resistance was not great. So fast had been our advance west of the Moselle that the Krauts had not had time to fortify the east bank against our crossing. By noon of March 14 the advance had gone well, so our guns were displaced closer to the river. Under a smoke screen the engineers were building a bridge, and by dusk it was completed. The artillery was ordered across, and then began another lurid evening. The road we started out on was a long, winding dirt trail running down the steep slope to the river. There we would hit the paved road parallel to the river, drive down it a couple of miles and then cross the recently completed pontoon bridge. Just before we started out, the Boche began to shell the west bank of the Moselle, down which we were to drive. Since they had been driven back during the day, their guns could not reach into the deep

Moselle valley, so they concentrated their fire on the west bank, which they could reach.

As I sat in my jeep in the gathering twilight, waiting to go down that blazing road, and listening to the report of the Kraut artillery and the whistle and crack of the shells, I shivered in the cold evening air (or was it from the cold?). It is hard to sit calmly and quietly by, waiting your turn to go down into a hell of bursting shells and dying men. As time went on the shelling increased in intensity, and then we started out. We tried to keep as wide an interval as possible between vehicles, but in the darkness we had to stay fairly close together so as not to get lost. As usual, we inched along slowly—oh, so slowly—often stopping for long, nerve-wracking waits. It really jars one's nervous system to sit for long periods in a stopped convoy while the enemy tries to shell the road one is on. The Krauts knew we would have to use this certain road, so they were doing their best to shoot it up. Since they were shooting "blind" in the darkness, their aim wasn't too good, and luckily for us most of their shells did not hit the road, but a lot of the rounds did come too close for comfort. Stabs of brilliant orange lighted the sky and hurtling steel fragments whistled through the air as the shells crashed close to us.

I sat hunched in my jeep, wondering if I'd ever get through this night. A shell ripped overhead and cracked not far away. A cry of "Medics!" went up, so I jumped off my jeep and ran up the road to the second truck in front of me, where an antiaircraft gunner had been hit. I went over to him quickly in the dark, but all I found was a minor arm wound, which I dressed the best I could. Then we went on again, starting and stopping, starting and stopping.

At the foot of the hill we passed through a little town which the Jerries were shooting into quite frequently. Of course, while I was in it the convoy stopped again, this time for about half an hour. I got off my jeep and stood beside a tank which was parked there. Every time a salvo of shells would scream in I'd crouch down in front of the tank for protection. Finally we started out again, reached the river and turned onto the paved road beside it. We were to drive upstream a couple of miles to the bridge. Now that the condition of the road was better the speed of the convoy began to increase.

Suddenly I thought I saw something looming up in front of us. I shouted a warning to Peter, who jerked the wheel to the left. Off the road we went, and for a sickening moment I thought we'd surely roll over into the river; but the jeep stopped short of the water. Wedl put it into reverse and somehow got it up the steep bank back onto the road. Then we saw that the "object" we had seen in front of us was a large white "splash" mark on the road where a shell had hit a short time before. That made us all the more anxious to "get along," so we started on again in a hurry.

After a while we reached the pontoon bridge, waited our turn to drive onto it and finally crossed it. The actual crossing was facilitated by a bit of artificial moonlight. When we reached the other side I breathed a sigh of relief, for at last we were safe. The enemy artillery could not reach us here, protected as we were by the high cliffs of the river valley. We drove down the river to Brodenbach, where we set up the command post and aid station in the town hall, and settled down for the rest of the night. I do not recall that we were unduly disturbed by enemy fire during the ensuing hours.

Early the next morning our infantry pushed out again against light opposition, so by midmorning we moved again in order to keep in close support. We wound our way up out of the deep river valley on a narrow dirt road with many horseshoe curves and hairpin turns. The gun trucks had great difficulty making the sharp turns and had to "seesaw" back and forth to get around them on this steep road. At last we reached a high plateau, drove a couple of miles from the river and went into position. The house we used for an aid station and command post was on fairly high ground and from that site we could see many little German towns on the surrounding hills. Some of the towns were being shelled by our artillery, and as I watched they were blanketed under the smoke of bursting shells.

Early the next morning we moved again. Soon after we had set up in our new location a couple of boys from the T.D.'s* came in

---

* Tank Destroyer Units.

to say that there was a badly wounded Boche soldier a couple of towns away, so I took my jeep and two men and followed them to the town. There I found an S.S. soldier with a compound fracture of his leg. We hated the S.S. troops, but of course we dressed his wound, splinted the leg and sent him back to the collecting company.

Later in the day we moved again. The town we moved the command post and aid station into, Hassenbach, had been heavily shelled by our artillery. One house, in the cellar of which had huddled an entire German family of eight or ten men, women and children, had been hit by an 8-inch shell, which had penetrated to the cellar and then exploded. The remains of the people lay scattered about in the ruins of the house in a ghastly display—a decapitated child, a legless man, the battered body of an infant covered by a bloody dress and diaper, an eviscerated young woman and so forth. I had no love for the Krauts, but such sights of civilian slaughter always sickened me. Of course, they are the very ones who "heiled" Hitler and started this whole mess, so they can blame themselves for it.

It was at Hassenbach that we lost two fine officers and I lost two good friends—Lieutenant Bauer, an air observer, and Lieutenant Hester, a cub pilot. A short distance outside of town a group of fanatical S.S. soldiers had set up a road block and were holding out to the end. In addition to their small arms they had several 88-mm. antitank guns and some 40-mm. antiaircraft guns. Our infantry hit this position, were stopped and called for artillery support. Lieutenants Hester and Bauer immediately took off in a cub to direct fire on the block. While flying low over the area their plane was hit by the Heinie ack-ack. A wing fell off and the plane plunged straight to the ground before either of the boys could get out. We saw the plane spin down, so I at once made preparations to try to get to the crash to give first aid, if either fellow was found to be still alive. Lieutenant Rizzo, our other cub pilot, reported from the air the site at which the plane had gone down—a very inaccessible spot in the center of a deep woods. To add to our difficulties, it was late in the afternoon and would soon be dark. It would be hard enough to find the wreckage in the daylight, and just about impossible to locate it in the dark.

Finally, in desperation, I asked Lieutenant Rizzo to fly me over the area to see for myself if anything could be done. We climbed into his cub and took off into the gathering gloom. I felt a bit uneasy to be soaring around up there right where the Jerries had knocked down a cub a short time before. I expected any second to be fired upon, but my fears were never realized. Suddenly, below us, we saw the wreckage of the other plane. We dropped low and cruised slowly around it, but there was no sign of life. Two battered bodies lay sprawled silently and grotesquely where they had been hurled from the plane. Sadly we flew back to Hassenbach, knowing that Bauer and Hester were dead. By now it was dark, but the next day an infantry patrol penetrated to the site of the crash. They confirmed my belief that both the boys had been killed when the plane hit the ground.

I'd like to make a few remarks here about these artillery spotter planes, which in my opinion were one of the best weapons the American army had. Most artillery battalions had two cub planes which went right along with the battalion, landing and taking off in any field or cow pasture near the guns. Weather permitting, one or the other (sometimes both) of these planes would be in the air all during daylight hours, observing enemy actions and directing artillery fire on likely targets. Each plane carried a pilot, an observer and a radio, but no armament at all. Through the radio the observer talked to the fire direction center and adjusted the fire of the artillery. In addition to directing the artillery, the cub planes were a tremendous help to the tanks and the infantry during rapid advances. While our long, fingerlike columns were rushing forward, the cubs would fly up and down and back and forth, reporting what was up ahead and warning our columns when there was danger from enemy attack on our flanks. The planes were not supposed to fly over enemy-held territory, but frequently they did, and were fired upon by German ack-ack. Now and then a Jerry fighter plane would make a pass at a cub, but then the cub would scoot down close to the ground, too low for the fighter to reach it. The

Germans hated these planes with a white-hot hate, for they knew the cubs were a chief reason for the accuracy of the devastating American artillery fire.

By this time the 4th Armored Division was running wild to our south. The day after we had secured our Moselle bridgehead they had crossed the river behind us, gone through our bridgehead and roared south to link up with the 7th Army. They were on their way now, cutting the German army in pieces. Our orders were to move south, cleaning up the area between the 4th Armored's southward thrust and the Rhine.

During its long slashes across Germany the 4th Armored Division used public-address loud speakers to advantage. When the columns came close to a town a tank with a loud speaker would move up close to town and a German interpreter would tell the villagers that if they would surrender without a fight their homes would be spared, but that if they resisted the village would be destroyed. Usually, white flags quickly appeared, and the tanks would roar on through the town without a fight, thus saving time and lives. Occasionally German troops (usually S.S.) would hold out in some village. Then a sharp fight would ensue, and the town would be left behind, a burning wreck.

The next morning a report came in that when a task force had taken a small town on the Rhine early that morning, they had found four wounded American soldiers in the town who had been left behind by the Jerries. I was asked to bring them in. Since my litter jeep would carry only three litters, I enlisted the aid of Captain Bolger, battalion surgeon of the 358th's third battalion. The town was 4 or 5 miles away, over almost impassable roads, and there were no American troops between there and Hassenbach. However, we set out in our two litter jeeps for the town, driving through dense, dark, silent forests and bumping over rough, rocky trails.

At last we came out on a high plateau on the west bank of the Rhine. It was a truly beautiful sight. Here the wide, majestic river flowed swiftly between high banks. Far below us was the river, and nestled along it were several pretty towns. We drove down a winding road into the village nearest us. There in the local hotel we found four rather badly wounded soldiers from the 358th infantry.

They had been captured several days before and had been quite well treated. When the Germans had retreated across the Rhine they could not take the wounded prisoners with them, so they left them there. We loaded them on our jeeps and started on the difficult road back. I also picked up a young German soldier captured by our boys and suspected of having diphtheria, and took him along, too. We got back at last, after a laborious trip.

That afternoon we moved south again, such movements continuing for several days until our division reached and took Bingen. Then the 90th swung east, following the Rhine,* and advanced rapidly toward Mainz, with only scattered resistance. Now, however, the *Luftwaffe* again put in an appearance, and we saw our first jet-propelled planes. These would come streaking in at tremendous speeds, suddenly slow down, drop their bombs and then race out of sight, with the ack-ack filling the sky with black puffs far behind the planes. A few days before we reached Mainz the *Luftwaffe* gave us a bad time. Our battalion had just moved into position one morning, and I was standing in a little house on the edge of town, looking over a site for my aid station. Suddenly I heard our antiaircraft cut loose, and in a moment the whine of diving planes and the soft whir of falling bombs. I had such a helpless, detached feeling as I stood in that little house. There was nothing I could do. If a bomb hit the house the flimsy roof would be no protection.

Then suddenly a cluster of antipersonnel bombs (the famous German butterfly bombs) hit in the center of one of our gun batteries a hundred yards from the house. The cry of "Medics!" went up, so out I ran. Above in the sky German planes were wheeling and weaving, and ahead of me were clouds of dust and smoke. Quickly the smoke drifted away, and I found the bleeding boys. We gave them first aid and sent them to the collecting company. Several times again the *Luftwaffe* returned, but we suffered no more casualties that day.

---

* This river runs generally north from the Swiss border to Mainz, where it makes a right-angle turn west for a short distance to Bingen. There it makes another right-angle turn and flows north again.

Late that afternoon we moved again, and set up the aid station and command post in another town. Across the street from the house we selected to use, a German air force soldier had shot his wife and then himself early that morning, shortly before our infantry came along. An ardent Nazi, the young man could not face life as he saw the evil Nazi system crashing around him, so he had killed himself and his pretty wife. I wonder if she knew she was going to die. She lay peacefully in bed, with an ugly, bloody hole behind her ear, and her husband lay on the floor with a big hole in his head and a Luger in his hand. Perhaps he shot her as she slept and then turned the gun on himself. Yes, the Germans were really beaten, and some could not face it.

After dark that night we were ordered to displace again. The infantry was about to enter Mainz, and we were moving to keep within range. This time I put the aid station in a German physician's office, one of the best arrangements I had thus far had. We were in a rather pretty little town that night. It had been debated whether to put the aid station and command post in that or in a solitary house a mile or two farther on down the road toward Mainz. Fortunately, the town was the place decided upon, for during the night about 75 bypassed Krauts who had been hiding in a near-by woods attacked the few American soldiers who had moved into that house. A pitched battle raged most of the night, resulting in heavy casualties on both sides. It was lucky that we had not located there, in the middle of it.

The next day, March 21, we moved into Finthen, a couple of miles from Mainz. Our guns were situated on the edge of town, and we had a whole house in the outskirts for the aid station. It was a nice setup for us, and we enjoyed our stay there while the infantry was mopping up in Mainz. Although the Heinies threw a few shells our way, it wasn't very bad.

For the past several weeks we had seen more and more liberated slave laborers. Thousands and thousands of them cluttered the roads—French, Poles, Russians, Czechs, Yugoslavs, Dutch, Belgians and so forth—men, women and children. They were pathetic sights as they trudged past us toward the rear—ragged, tired, starved and sickly, carrying their worldly possessions on their backs or pulling them along in rickety carts. Yet they were unspeakably happy and grateful to be free again. Most of them had fared miserably as German slaves. They had been worked hard and had been poorly fed and sometimes cruelly treated. What a horrible system the Germans had built up! Most of these unhappy creatures had been crowded into dirty, dingy, unpainted wooden shacks, surrounded by barbed-wire fences. These had been their homes for several long years.

PART THREE

Chapter Thirteen

ACROSS THE RHINE

*M*AINZ HAD FALLEN AND THE LAND WEST OF the Rhine had been cleared of enemy troops. About noon on March 23 our battalion commander called us together for a meeting. He told us that the Fifth Infantry Division had crossed the Rhine in assault boats south of us near Nierstein early that morning and was advancing well. The plan was for the Third Army to pour through that bridgehead, but for a change the battle-weary 90th was not to spearhead the way. We were to be preceded by six or eight divisions, but then, an hour later, just as we expected, the plans were changed, and the old 90th was ordered to cross the Rhine as soon as possible behind the 5th. We were to be the second division across and were to expand the bridgehead eastward, so that we would be up to our ears in blood again. Our infantry moved out right away and crossed in boats, but since the artillery had to wait for a bridge to be built, we did not move until the next day.

About 0800 we left Finthen and moved south 10 or 15 miles to an assembly area near Selzen, a couple of miles west of the Rhine, keeping a weather eye out all the way for the *Luftwaffe*. Now that American troops had crossed the Rhine, the *Luftwaffe* was making a final desperate effort to stem the tide. Early in the afternoon we set out from the assembly area for the crossing. Faces were a little grim, nerves were tense and tempers were short that day. "Just one more river to cross," we said, "and then maybe this whole thing will soon be over." We knew that Jerry would fight hard to contain our bridgehead, but we also knew that we had the overwhelming power to steam-roller him. Before long—maybe in another month or two—Germany would be overrun. But that knowledge, while it cheered us, also tightened already overstrung nerves. We had lasted out almost 10 months of the hell of battle—wouldn't it be ironic to be killed now that victory was in sight?

"Why don't these Krauts quit?" we kept asking. "They're whipped and they all know it. Why don't they stop this foolishness? Their hope of victory is long gone, and their continuation of this bloodshed and misery and destruction is criminal!"

So, thinking these things, we inched along the road to Nierstein and the pontoon bridge across the Rhine. Our long column of trucks and guns, stretching over miles of dusty roads, moved along exasperatingly slowly. On either side of us marched a line of soldiers, trudging toward the front. Above us in the sky we saw occasional "dogfights" as our air corps drove off enemy planes attempting to bomb the bridge. The afternoon wore on, and soon it was evening. About dark we entered Nierstein and snaked through it to the river. What a congested place it was and what confusion! It seemed as if the whole Third Army was trying to cross the river at once. Tanks, trucks, men and guns congested every street and road leading to the crossing site. The bridge was well protected against air attack, for both banks of the river above and below it were lined with antiaircraft guns—quadruple 50's and Bofors guns—and farther back on each side were many batteries of 90-mm. antiaircraft guns.

A short time before I was to drive onto the pontoon bridge our column ahead of me was broken to allow several thousand German prisoners to be run back across the river, so I sat in the darkness watching the shadowy figures of the prisoners trot by us toward the rear, and hoping I would get over the river before the *Luftwaffe* returned. At last the prisoners were all across and our column started again. Then it happened. Just before my jeep started down the ramp to the bridge, over came the *Luftwaffe*. Our antiaircraft guns opened up with a deafening roar. Above us was an interlacing canopy of bullets and exploding 40-mm. shells, while higher up burst the 90-mm. shells. The sky was ablaze over our heads with thousands of red tracer bullets and flashing ack-ack shell-bursts. It was light enough to read by (but I had no desire to read, for some reason!). No plane could have come through that steel screen and none tried. The German pilots dropped their bombs from high up, missing the bridge by a mile. While all this was going on we drove across the bridge as fast as we could, breathing a prayer of thanks when we got over safely.

However, our troubles were not over, for we had to find the rest of the battalion somewhere over there in the darkness. As I bounced along in my jeep, straining my eyes to follow the truck ahead of me, I hoped that whoever was in the lead vehicle knew where he was going. If he did not, we might blunder into the German lines. The countryside was dotted with burning towns; the dirt roads were clogged with men and machines; above us buzzed many enemy planes looking for profitable targets; 90-mm. ack-ack shells cracked and flashed as they shot toward the planes; and over all was a feeling of utter confusion. Each town we had to go through was a bottleneck, for the narrow streets further slowed down the many convoys trying to get through. About 2300 hours our convoy stopped again, this time putting me in the middle of a blazing town.

"Our artillery surely shot up this place," I thought to myself, but about then I was told that the *Luftwaffe* had caused the damage when they had bombed it about 20 minutes before. After I heard that, the half-hour we sat there waiting to move seemed like an eternity, but finally we moved on again before the *Luftwaffe* paid a return visit.

A little later we made contact with the rest of the battalion and turned off toward our bivouac area for the night. Shortly before we got there the convoy was held up again by a traffic jam—jeeps, trucks, tanks, half-tracks, guns and so forth, lined up bumper to bumper on both sides of the road. I got off the jeep to stretch my legs and see what was going on. Jerry planes had been droning over us all night so far, and hence I paid little attention to another one approaching us, until I heard the soft whir of falling bombs. Then I hit the dirt—but fast! The plane had dropped a stick of butterfly bombs, which hit a hundred yards or so away from the road. I lay pressed to the ground as the bombs roared, and steel fragments screamed through the air. Then I arose a little shakily and found that no one had been hurt. I'm glad that bombardier's aim was off.

Soon afterward we found the battalion's bivouac area and got settled for the night. We put the aid station in one of the wooden barracks of some sort of labor camp. The command post was in another barracks near us. The camp was poorly camouflaged by a thin growth of trees, and the wooden buildings would give little protection against attack by enemy planes. We spent an uneasy night as many German planes droned over us, some of them seeming to be low enough to scrape the trees; but none of them attacked us. Of course, our antiaircraft did not open fire. We had learned early by bitter experience that at night it is better not to disclose one's position by firing at enemy planes unless they see you and attack you.

The next day the Fourth Armored Division crossed the Rhine behind us, roared through our bridgehead and swept into enemy territory. Our infantry took Darmstadt without much trouble and then turned north toward the Main River. Darmstadt, like all German cities, was a ghost town—a city of the dead and of total destruction. We passed dozens of enemy antiaircraft batteries ringing the city, their guns either destroyed or pointing parallel to the ground, for they had been used as a last desperate effort to stop our tanks and infantry. During the day we displaced several times in order to keep up with the infantry advance, for the boys were going ahead against little opposition now. Our last move was made after dark, and was a long one. Soon after we got started the *Luft-waffe* again attacked the pontoon bridges over the Rhine. Although we were several miles from there, I felt uneasy. The flares, even at that distance, lighted us with a ghastly half-light. The ground rumbled with the noise of falling bombs, the roar of aircraft engines and the explosions of ack-ack guns and shells. I was afraid that some of the enemy pilots, finding the bridge area "too hot," might spot our convoy and attack us; but that did not occur.

The German populace realized that the war had been lost long ago, and greeted us with a resigned, stoical air. Every town and village, under orders from the Nazi party, had constructed heavy road blocks of huge logs and stones on each road into town. An opening was left in each road block, to be closed as we approached. The road blocks were then to be defended to the death by the *Volkssturm*.* The civilians realized that further resistance was useless, and the *Volkssturm* never functioned against us except in isolated instances. After we once got rolling across Germany I never once saw one of these road blocks closed. So fast was our advance that they had no time to close them. As soon as the S. S. troops and Nazi officials in the town had fled, the local *Volkssturm* would disband and quietly await the arrival of the Americans.

The next night we stayed in some rickety barracks at a former enemy searchlight and aircraft listening station—one of the many such stations comprising part of the elaborate antiaircraft protection around Frankfurt. To the northwest we heard the din of terrific cannonading as the Sixth Armored and Fifth Infantry Divisions battered their way into the ruins of Frankfurt. The Germans depressed the many antiaircraft guns around the city against the advancing Americans, and fought viciously from gun to gun. During the night our infantry crossed the Main in assault boats east of Frankfurt against almost no opposition. The engineers put in a pontoon bridge, and the next night the artillery rolled across. Farther east the Fourth Armored crossed the river and started off toward Fürth to the northeast with the 90th following behind. Soon great columns of German prisoners began to stream back as the Fourth Armored cut deeper into the Reich. Now we began to see many more thousands of slave laborers—men, women and children of all the oppressed nations of Europe. They wandered aimlessly around, literally by the thousands, jubilant at being free. Of course, there were many cases in which the newly liberated slaves helped themselves to belongings of their former masters, but in general they were far more orderly than I expected. These days we moved fast, frequently going into position three or four times a day, but seldom doing any firing.

---

* The "People's Army."

Our advance was to the northeast, and so fast was it that we had little time to clean out the areas we passed through. In one place near the town of Stockem we overlooked a large force of S. S. troops hiding in some woods. After we had gone by, they retook Stockem, cut our main line of communication, captured a hospital of the Fourth Armored Division, raided supply columns and in general terrorized our rear area. For some days it was quite dangerous to travel around in the rear, and all supply trains were convoyed by tanks. However, in time all the loose enemy were rounded up by the 71st Division, which was "mopping up" behind us.

Chapter Fourteen

THE DASH ACROSS GERMANY

*L*ATE IN THE AFTERNOON OF MARCH 31 WE STOPPED in the village of Sandhof, where we spent the next day and night. The ensuing day was Sunday, April 1, Easter. I went to a nice Easter service in a local church, held by our chaplain and attended by many of our soldiers. It seemed strange to be taking time out of the war to remember the resurrection of the Prince of Peace. How far the world drifts from His teachings! The day was quiet, but not easy on the nerves. We had been told that the next day the Fourth Armored and the 90th Divisions were to start east, spearheading a drive to split Germany in two and to link up with the Russians. We spent the day going over our vehicles and supplies. We were to throw away all unnecessary things, lighten our loads to a minimum, stock up on gasoline and a week's rations and get ready for another wild dash. It was a quite exciting prospect, and yet a bit disquieting. We were anxious to finish up the war, but to our war-weary minds such a task as that before us was not pleasant. However, before we started, plans were changed and our scheduled dash did not take place. Instead we continued a steady but slower advance eastward. During the night of April 1 an ammunition truck of "A" Battery caught fire and all night long the shells stored on it exploded one or two at a time. It was thought that a German soldier hiding near by had sneaked in after dark close enough to fire a *Panzerfaust* (a German antitank weapon) into the truck.

About dawn the next morning, April 2, we pulled out and started east under cloudy skies. Some time along in the middle of the morning, as our convoy slowly wound over the roads, I glanced up from my seat on my jeep at the sound of airplane engines. Suddenly, out of the clouds swooped six planes, flying quite low.

"Glad to see that our air corps is on the job," I thought absent-mindedly, but almost simultaneously I realized that the fuselage of those planes looked long and a bit painfully familiar, and that they were Messerschmitt ME 109's. At the same moment they "peeled off" and came diving at our convoy. Our .50 caliber machine guns opened up with a deafening roar, the trucks hauling the 40 mm. Bofors antiaircraft guns pulled off the road to get the guns in firing position, all vehicles stopped and men spilled off them into the ditches and fields. For a few moments I stood beside my jeep in strange fascination watching a Messerschmitt ME 109 diving toward me.

"Look at that stream of tracer bullets!" I thought, but then I noticed that they were coming *toward* me and were from the plane and not from an antiaircraft gun shooting at the plane, as I had first supposed.

I broke all records getting away from that road. I raced into a field and flung myself into a plot of ground enclosed by a crumbling stone fence. There I lay behind the fence while the Kraut planes roared up and down, strafing the convoy. The attack didn't last long, for our antiaircraft fire was too intense. A couple of the planes were hit, and the others fled. Then I looked around me and noticed for the first time that I had taken refuge in an old Jewish cemetery. Many of the Hebrew-inscribed stones had fallen down; the entire plot was overgrown with weeds, bushes and brambles, and the stone fence was in ruins, for this was anti-Semitic Germany, where Jewish cemeteries were not kept up. I stood up and walked back to my jeep, thanking the Jews of Germany for having aided me. No one had been hurt and the convoy had received little damage, so we started on again as best we could under the tense strain, with one eye watching the sky.

The rest of the day we moved ahead rapidly, stopping now and then to fire our guns in support of the infantry when they hit occasional pockets of resistance. We saw a few more Heinie planes, but none bothered our column. It rained during the afternoon, so we were thoroughly wet and uncomfortable as we drove along. However, we got an adequate house for the aid station and command post for the night, so we could at least get dry.

The next morning a Polish slave laborer came to us to ask for aid for some injured slave laborers in the next town. Wedl and I drove up there and found three rather badly wounded persons—a Polish woman, a Polish man and a Russian man. All had been shot by retreating S.S. troops a few days before. They lived with a large crowd of other slave laborers in a barbed-wire enclosed camp, in miserable, dirty, unpainted wooden barracks. The slaves had been liberated the day before, and were a happy lot. We loaded the wounded onto our litter jeep and evacuated them.

Early in the afternoon we moved again. As we drove along the road we saw the bodies of quite a few dead American and German soldiers in the ditches. In one spot, where one of our tanks had been hit, lay a group of four horribly burned corpses. I always did hate to see dead American boys, but at this late date in the war it hurt me more than ever. We knew the Germans were done for, so it seemed so useless for our lads to have to keep on dying. Sometimes I'd walk over to a fallen boy, look down at his still face, read his name on his "dog tags," look at his blood-soaked uniform, see the wedding ring on the finger of his outstretched hand and wonder about his loved ones so far away who were yet to receive that telegram from the War Department.

Just before we reached the town where we were to stop for the night we heard the sound of heavy rifle and machine-gun fire a short distance off the road to our left. We didn't stop to investigate, but later we learned that a hundred or so well dug-in S.S. troops had elected to fight it out there. After a sharp battle, our infantry cleaned them out, and a little later I saw the prisoners. Most of these S.S. troops had been killed, but about 30 had surrendered. They were a motley crew—those "supermen."

About a mile or so behind us was a little town in which were set up the headquarters of the 358th Infantry Regiment and Collecting Company B (the medical collecting company to which I normally evacuated my casualties). After I got my aid station set up I drove back to establish contact with the collecting company, talked with Captain Gordon and the other medical officers there and returned to my station. A short time later I heard the buzz of planes and the rattle of ack-ack, so I knew the planes were German. I ran to the door, heard the heavy roar of a terrific explosion in the distance and saw a huge cloud of smoke rising from the town I had just left. At first I was puzzled, wondering how a fighter plane could have dropped a bomb capable of such an explosion and if perhaps the Germans had a new, much more powerful explosive. Soon I learned the answer. The enemy planes had suddenly appeared over the town. One got away, but one was shot down and crashed into a house on the outskirts of the town. Just before it crashed the pilot jettisoned a bomb which, by a strange quirk of fate, hit a German railway car sitting on a track in the town. The railway car had been loaded with TNT, and it was this tremendous explosion which we had heard and seen.

Soon I got a hurry call to come help out in the stricken town, so I loaded some of my men on my jeep and started. When we got to the house the falling plane had hit we were stopped by some frantic German civilians, so we gave first aid to some badly injured people there and then drove into the town. What a shambles! The center of town, where the box car of TNT had stood, was gone. I don't think a house in town was undamaged, and all buildings near the explosion had collapsed. Civilians ran screaming through the streets seeking their families or carrying bleeding children in their arms. Dazed and bleeding soldiers wandered around. Some soldiers and many civilians were killed and buried in the ruins. The building housing the collection company had been damaged, and almost every member of the company had been injured, some lightly and some seriously. One medical officer lost an eye, and Captain Gordon, Captain Rose and Lieutenant Myers were all cut by flying glass and débris. My men and I went to work caring for the stream of injured soldiers and German civilians who came in, and we worked until after dark. On our way back we stopped to look at the wreckage of the crashed plane and the charred body of the pilot.

The next day we moved on again—rapidly, as usual. We had the unusual experience of being fired upon by American artillery this day. Our guns had just gone into position on one stop, when a shell hit near the houses occupied by the aid station and command post. Then another, and another. Some artillery was obviously adjusting its fire on us and getting ready to blast our position. The shells came from our rear, so we wondered if they might be from some German guns by-passed in the woods around us, for we had advanced too rapidly to clean out any woods. However, it was soon discovered that the fire came from an American 155-mm. howitzer battalion behind us. They were immediately informed in no uncertain terms of their mistake, and the fire ceased before we suffered any casualties. The same day we overran and liberated a prison camp of British soldiers and one of Italian prisoners.

We were now near the town of Merkers, and all around us were salt mines. We heard from some of the Italian prisoners of war that the Germans had hidden money and loot in some of the mines. The 357th Infantry investigated this tip, and located 100 tons of gold bullion, 5,000,000,000 German marks, 2,000,000 American dollars, 2,000 famous paintings and hundreds of pieces of sculpture. The 357th was left behind to guard this treasure for a while.

The next day we entered the town of Bad Liebsstein, formerly a German health resort, but now housing eight or ten enemy military hospitals. It seemed strange to see enemy soldiers (medics) walking freely around the streets. I went through one of the hospitals, being escorted by a staff of heel-clicking bowing officers. Some of the badly wounded soldiers scowled at me, but that was all. Of course, the hospitals were in dire need of supplies.

We were on our way again the next day, passing through many towns and seeing thousands more slave laborers and their miserable camps. Late in the afternoon we passed through Zella-Mehlis, and went into position several miles east of town. In Zella-Mehlis was located the famous Walther Arms Factory. The factory was loaded with weapons, so we took our share of souvenir P-38 and .32-caliber pistols.

The next day we retraced our steps through Zella-Mehlis, drove south a few miles to Suhl and then turned east again. We were advancing almost at will these days. The German armed forces had disintegrated, although we still hit pockets of resistance here and there. When we did, the artillery would shell the town in question, and then the infantry would move in to mop up; so we left a trail of shattered and burning villages in our wake. It was a pathetic sight to drive through a burning town and watch the civilians trying to extinguish the fires and to save what they could from their flaming and shattered homes, but we had little time to spend in sympathizing with their troubles. We were too intent upon the job at hand, and we were too occupied with our own hopes and fears. We now could see the end of the conflict, and more than ever we longed to return home unhurt. During the dark days of Normandy, when death was so close at hand every minute, I had resigned myself to the probability that my lot was to die in Europe. But now, although we had obviously won the war, the fighting was still going on and many men were yet to be killed. I think all of us felt the increasing tension, and hoped for peace before our names were added to the growing casualty lists.

As we advanced across Germany we saw many of their *Autobahns,* the four-to-six-lane superhighways which criss-crossed the country—real dream roads. It was interesting to see how they had used stretches of these for their air corps. Since all known German airfields were targets for our bombers, the Jerries figured out a rather clever scheme. They'd select a place where the *Autobahn* passed through a heavy forest and then emerged for a straight, clear stretch for a mile or two. During the day they'd keep their planes hidden in the forest, and at night they'd taxi out on the highway and use it for a runway.

On April 12 the battalion moved to the outskirts of a little town called Pleasant. Since we were moving so fast and were to be there only a short time and then go on again, we did not set up an aid station or a command post. We pulled our trucks off the road in the yard of a lumber company just outside the town. A few hundred yards down the road was another little town on a hillside, which, unknown to us, our troops had not yet entered. As I stood by my jeep in the lumber yard, several tanks and tank destroyers loaded with infantry roared by toward that town. When they reached the edge of the town they were fired upon by a few enemy troops, so immediately the doughboys leaped from the vehicles and deployed, and the tanks and tank destroyers swung about for action. I stood in the road fascinated. The tanks and tank destroyers let go with their 76-mm. guns and their .50-caliber machine guns while the doughboys advanced toward the town. Houses crumbled under the pounding, débris flew into the air, flames spurted up and over all rose a cloud of smoke and dust. When the riflemen had reached the town the tanks ceased firing, and then lumbered on through it when the enemy had been driven out. The doughboys jumped back onto their steel steeds and roared off over the hills, leaving the dying town behind.

A little later we were ordered to move on again, so we started off. It began to rain and then to pour, and what a wet, miserable ride we had! I wore a raincoat, but the driving rain beating on us in the open jeep seeped through every crevice and soon I was wet and cold. On and on we drove, hour after hour, shivering and uncomfortable. Finally, just before dark, we stopped for the night in a little town, and the firing batteries went into position around the town.

We had picked up a German radio for the use of our medical section, so every evening, after we had stopped for the night, we'd hook it into the generator giving light for the command post and listen to it. It was interesting and amusing to tune in on the few remaining enemy stations in operation and have Peter Wedl translate the propaganda. Usually they'd alternate stirring martial music with passionate speeches by screaming orators, flaying "American barbarians" and exhorting the faithful to stand by the *Führer*. Then, of course, Lord Haw-Haw* had not yet been captured, and was still giving his "Views of the News," spewing out his lies about the "Jewish capitalists" and "Russian Bolsheviks:" At this late hour the Göbbels† propaganda mill was having trouble, but it still functioned.

---

* William Joyce. He was hanged by the British at London on January 3, 1946.
† He and his wife, after poisoning their children, killed themselves in the ruins of the *Reichskanzlei* in Berlin on the night of April 29–30, 1945.

The next evening, when we stopped for the night, we took over two rooms in a German house for the aid station. The owner of the house, a small, sad-looking man, walked around watching us, but said nothing. A little later one of my boys called me in a hurry to the attic, where the fellow had hanged himself. I found the limp body already cold, and the face purple, so all I could do was to cut him down. I wonder why he took his life—fear? Despair? Guilt? Insanity? I'll never know. We notified the *Bürgermeister*, and the man's relatives came and hauled off the body in a little hand cart. It was incongruous to watch the little cart bouncing over the rough street and to see a lifeless arm, hanging out the side from under a blanket, waving up and down with every bump of the wheels.

A few days later, on about the 15th, the 358th Infantry took Hof, a city only a few miles from Czecho-Slovakia. The artillery went into position in a little town on the southern outskirts, where we rested for a couple of days. Hof had been heavily damaged, but not destroyed, by bombing, shelling and street fighting. While I was there I visited a German airfield just outside the city, climbing over the numerous old training planes and bombers parked around.

About midnight the first night we were in this position, Lieutenant Leslie Olbetter, one of our cub pilots, came into the aid station to ask me if I would go see a seriously ill Dutch woman. I got up out of my bed roll, put on my shoes and jacket, woke Wedl and the three of us started out in my jeep. We drove down the dark, empty road to Hof (wondering how safe we were from attack), into the outskirts of town, past still-burning buildings and to a settlement of foreign workers. I found the ill woman in one of the small cottages, where she lived with her 15-year-old daughter. She was a Dutch woman whose husband had been killed by the Gestapo and who had been brought to Germany four years before to work for German officers. She had undergone appendectomy in a Hof hospital a few days before, and since she was a "foreigner," she had been turned out of the hospital a couple of days afterward, to get along as best she could.

Her incision had broken open and she was in critical condition. She had peritonitis and was much dehydrated; she had a high fever and was suffering considerable pain. Thin, watery pus was draining from her wound. I did what I could for her with sulfa-diazine given by mouth, sulfanilamide powder sifted into the wound, the injection of morphine and the giving of a few instructions. The next day I loaded her onto my litter jeep and took her to the collecting station for evacuation to a hospital. She was overjoyed when I told her she was going to an American hospital, for she had tearfully told me that she'd rather die than go to a German hospital again. Apparently she had been badly treated.

While we were around Hof, the Third Battalion of the 358th Infantry sent a task force into Czecho-Slovakia, simply to cross the border. Our boys suffered no casualties, took 36 prisoners and returned safely. The next day we started out again, south this time instead of east. The Germans expected the Third Army to keep on rolling east into Czecho-Slovakia, but General Patton swung his forces on a right angle and started south instead. The 90th was now the left-flank division of the Third Army, and our combat team was on the left flank of the division front, with the Czech border as our left boundary. We were advancing southward fast, and we also had to worry about protecting the ever-lengthening left flank of the Third Army from enemy attack and infiltration, a not-easy task. Fortunately for us, the Krauts were in no position to launch an attack. They were washed up and knew it, and were mostly trying to save their own hides.

On the 21st of April we picked up two American soldiers who had escaped from German captivity, and their miserable condition made our blood boil. They were thin, starved, beaten, sick and infested with lice; and were weak, tired and listless. They had lived through hell, and their haunted eyes, ragged clothes and broken bodies showed it. One of the boys had been with the 28th Division and the other had been with the 106th Division, and both had been captured four months before, during the Ardennes breakthrough, with thousands of others of our boys. Immediately after they had been captured their overcoats had been taken from them and they had then been marched 100 miles in snow and howling blizzards. They were put to work in mines and driven and beaten unmercifully. Since the fact that they had been captured had never been reported by the German authorities, they had not received any Red Cross prisoner-of-war packages. They had been fed only weak soup and a little bread.

When we had crossed the Rhine and started our dash across the *Reich,* all these prisoners had been herded together and marched eastward as fast as possible. As the weary men would fall by the road from exhaustion, emaciation and disease, the brutal guards would shoot them where they lay. We were fast catching up with the pitiful procession, and these two men had managed to hide in a woods, where they were when they heard the sound of our guns. They waited in the woods until we came along, and then they came out. They were almost too weak to walk, so I took them back to the collecting company for evacuation to a hospital. A few days later other units of our division caught up with the remnants of the group of prisoners. Most of them were more dead than alive, but they were all soon back in American hospitals. We could only hope they would achieve a return to good health and happiness.

During the past few weeks we had left a trail of shattered towns in our wake. Many a night I stood outside my aid station watching the flaming buildings in that particular town be consumed, and seeing the glow in the sky of other burning towns; and many a day I choked in the heavy, smoke-filled streets of a dying village as we drove through it. Well, the Heinies still preferred to fight, so their homes would continue to be shelled and burned. It was better to shoot up these towns than to lose a lot of our men by trying to take them entirely by storm.

Our own casualties were light these days, but I was busy much of the time caring for ill and injured civilians and foreign slave laborers. What a pathetic sight they were—this backwash of a cruel war. I saw many patients every day—with compound fractures of the skull, gangrenous legs, infected sores, compound fractured arms and legs and pale, sickly, undernourished children, tuberculous men and women, scabetic and lousy people by the dozen and so forth. There were almost no civilian physicians available, and their medical supplies were nil. I did what I could for the sufferers— civilian and slave alike—although sometimes I felt like refusing aid to the Germans when I saw how badly the foreign slaves had fared at the hands of their formerly arrogant "masters." However,

I never refused aid to any person. After all, I am a physician, and so I made not-a-few long day trips and dangerous night journeys to help some suffering Europeans.

On April 23 American troops took the little Bavarian town of Flossenbürg and liberated the infamous Flossenbürg concentration camp. We heard about its horrors, and so the next morning Peter Wedl, Major Lippard, Lieutenant Kean and I drove over to see it. I'll never forget that visit. It was only one of dozens of concentration camps in Germany, but what a cesspool of suffering and torture and human degradation! One who has not seen it cannot visualize it in his mind, and I am sure that one who has not lived through the never-ending days and nights of terror in such a place cannot possibly comprehend a fraction of its misery. Flossenbürg normally held 10,000 to 15,000 tortured souls, but when we got to it all but 1,500 of the inmates had been herded farther inland.

I have never before or since seen such wild, delirious joy as that shown by these pitiful 1,500 at their deliverance. Great holes had been torn in the barbed-wire fences by the madly happy prisoners when they first saw American troops. Not a few prisoners were seriously hurt by the barbed wire, but they didn't care. Liberty had been long in coming and was not to be delayed another instant. The camp had been built on the side of a hill and in a little valley. It was surrounded by an inner 10-foot-high fence of barbed wire and an outer 12 or 14-foot fence of electrified barbed wire. At intervals there were concrete towers for guards with machine guns. And of course at night the outside had been patrolled by vicious S.S. guards with equally vicious police dogs.

I could not immediately comprehend all I saw, but slowly I began to understand the incredibly cruel plan of the Germans, and their fiendish efficiency and meticulous detail. Adjoining the camp was an airplane factory, where the prisoners worked long hours six days a week making parts for German planes. They were fed only watery soup twice a day, and as they died of starvation, overwork, beatings or tortures, their wasted corpses were burned and new victims were sent in to take their places in the production line. In the four years of Flossenbürg's operation, between 60,000 and 100,000 miserable souls died there in agony (between 35 and 60 a day).

It should be remembered by all Americans that it was here that 15 of our brave, gallant paratroopers were hanged one Christmas Eve. Their "crime"? They had escaped from a prison camp and they were American paratroopers (whom the Krauts feared and hated). At the war crimes trial in Nürnberg it was testified that at Flossenbürg Concentration Camp on Christmas Eve, December 24, 1944, 15 American paratroopers were hanged by the S.S. beside gaily decorated Christmas trees, at a sadistic "Christmas party" for the inmates, who were compelled to watch the exhibition.

The first place I visited at the camp was the crematory. It was a well-built brick building with a cement floor and a large, efficient iron cremating furnace. Although the camp had been liberated, inmates were still dying in large numbers in spite of all we did for them, and their bodies were being burned as before, as a sanitary measure. I opened the door of the blazing furnace and there inside I saw three corpses sizzling and burning. In a room beside the furnace room I saw 15 or 20 naked bodies stacked up like cordwood, ready for their turn in the furnace. All the corpses looked almost like skeletons, so thin and emaciated were they. It was a weird place—the crackling furnace and the naked corpses with their lolling heads and stiff arms and legs. A little hand-operated "railway" (such as those often seen in mines) ran from all over the camp to the crematory to expedite the flow of the dead to the flames. Each morning on "rounds" those who had died during the night were collected, dumped into the carts, and pushed to the furnace. The crematory operators were three prisoners, all of them German political prisoners, whose spirits had long since been broken by their masters. They did their odious task in stolid silence. One of them had spent nine years in concentration camps. Had we not taken Flossenbürg when we did, these men would have worked here until they "knew too much," and then the S.S would have killed them, tossed them into the furnace, and selected three more for the job. I hated to see the crematory still in operation now that we were in command, but what else could be done with the many who were still dying? Incidentally, the Germans had used the ashes from here as fertilizer.

On six days the prisoners worked in the airplane factory, but the seventh day was a special day of torture and humiliation. On this day they were subjected to all the cruelties and indecencies the S.S. guards could think of. They had to clean out latrines with their hands, they had to crawl long distances dragging full latrine buckets with their teeth, they had to roll and grovel in the dust before their "lords and masters," they were beaten senseless, they were hung up by their hands, they were kicked in the testicles by laughing guards until they collapsed from pain, and on and on. I talked with many of the prisoners through Peter Wedl as an interpreter, and all the stories were the same.

From the crematory in one corner of the camp, we walked over to the center of the camp and looked into some of the barracks where the prisoners had lived. They were bare, drab, one-story frame buildings, with narrow three-decker wooden bunks. The bunks had only boards—no springs or mattresses, or even straw— and on each bunk, hardly wide enough for one man to sleep, three prisoners had been crowded each night.

All around us were the happy, incredulous prisoners, hardly daring to believe that they really were free again. They gathered around us, with tears of joy and gratitude in their eyes. They were all so terribly thin and emaciated, and almost too weak to walk. Their ragged blue and white striped prison clothes hung loosely on their bony frames. Their backs and arms were scarred from the many lashings they had endured, and some of them were deformed and crippled by their abuses. Of course, all had shaven heads and a blue prisoner number tattooed on the left forearm. Many had broken under the horrors, and their spirits had been crushed completely. They wandered around like cringing, beaten dogs, unable to comprehend that their bondage was over. They were the living dead. For them the joy of life had been extinguished under the heel of the *Schutzstaffel*. The prisoners were from almost every country of Europe—Russia, Poland, Czecho-Slovakia, France, Greece, Belgium, Holland, Germany and even Spain. They were all mixed up together, but some had been treated better than others by the diabolic S.S. guards, in order to stir up hatred and jealousies among the prisoners and to promote rivalries in grovel-ling before the guards for "favors," such as fewer beatings. The S.S. guards had been the high and mighty masters, and the unfortu-nate inmates had been at their absolute mercy and caprice. Every time one of these devils passed a prisoner, the inmate had to stop, snatch off his cap, and bow his head in reverence. If he was a frac-tion of a second too slow in doing this, he probably would be beaten senseless.

I talked with not a few of the prisoners—a Greek boy who had been here since he was 14 years old, a Belgian physician whose "crime" was refusing to give the names of Belgian underground members to the Gestapo, a German who had disagreed with Hit-ler, Russians who had been guerrilla fighters, Poles who happened to be Jews and so forth. What revolting stories of fiendish brutal-ity they told us.

Next I saw the camp "hospital," a large, barn-like building with straw on the floor. Here the dying were brought to end their miser-able existence. The sick were simply dumped on the straw, where they lay in their own vomitus and excreta if they were too weak to move. Each morning the dead were collected, but the rest of the time the living lay intermingled with those who had already died. The camp physician had been a sadistic S.S. doctor who had experi-mented on many of the inmates and had mutilated hundreds. Cas-trations, unnecessary amputations, gastrectomies "just for fun," and so forth, were common. He died of typhus shortly before we got there, so he never felt our justice. I longed to do something for the living, who looked up at me from the filthy straw, but all I could do was to tell them that soon American medical units would be here to care for them. I could not stay there long, for I had to accompany my own unit. The war was still on. Before long, however, our Medical Corps did take over the care of these men, but in spite of all their care, many of the unfortunates continued to die every day for many days. There was much typhus among these men.

Then I saw a large underground room where political prisoners were shot and where others were hung from hooks in the ceiling and tortured. At night the listening inmates could hear the muffled screams of the suffering and the pistol shots of the executioners.

The camp grounds were neat and clean, with characteristic German orderliness. The barracks were all laid out in exact rows and were built just alike.

Lastly, I saw one of the beautiful houses in which the S.S. guards, both men and women, had lived. There were 8 or 10 fine, large homes built on the hills around the camp. They were exquisitely furnished and very comfortable. Here the brutal S.S. guards had lived in luxury and revelry with their S.S. women. There were no female inmates at Flossenbürg, but these women had been there to keep the male guards happy. The S.S. did not take marriage seriously, and all the men had mistresses—the S.S. women. The prisoners told me that these women were more cruel and sadistic and blood-thirsty than were even the men. All the S.S., however, both men and women, were without mercy or honor or conscience.

When we left Flossenbürg to rejoin our unit we drove back over a dirt road through the woods, along which were strewn old coats, worn blankets, dirty comforts and so forth. I knew what had happened, and from this mute evidence I could reconstruct the pathetic story. A few days before about 13,000 of the prisoners from the Flossenbürg camp (all except the 1500 we had seen there) had been herded out onto this road and started marching to the southeast, away from our advancing troops. Up and down along the pitiful column had strode the S.S. guards, swinging their clubs freely on all who lagged, and spraying with their machine pistols all who fell by the wayside. The weary, weak, sick prisoners had started out carrying a coat or a blanket for protection from the damp, cold nights, but before they had trudged a mile their extra burdens had proved too heavy for their wasted bodies to carry, so they had tossed them aside and struggled on without them. I wonder how many of those 13,000 are alive today.

We got back to the battalion in time to move with them south to Pleystein and then to Burkhardreuth. The next day we moved to Schönsee, which was only a mile or so from the border of Czecho-Slovakia. When Lieutenant Mann, one of our artillery liaison officers with the 358th Infantry, asked me if I would like to drive across the border with him to a nearby Czech town to contact the first battalion, I jumped at the chance. I was anxious to get into Czecho-Slovakia, and since the division was proceeding south in Germany parallel to the Czech west boundary, it looked as if I might not get into that country. (Later, of course, we did.)

Some of the forces of the 358th were proceeding south across the Czech border as a screen for our left flank, and it was these whom Lieutenant Mann wanted to reach. We met no troops on our drive between towns, and so it was a good feeling to see some American soldiers as we entered the Czech town. I hated to think of driving around blindly in enemy territory. The people of the village were friendly, but not too demonstrative, a fact which puzzled me until later I realized that although I had actually been in Czecho-Slovakia, the territory we entered had been the old Sudetenland, where the inhabitants were pro-German.

On April 26 we moved to Trefelstein, where we stayed for four days. It was obvious to all of us that the European war was winding up, but no one dared guess how many more weeks we would be fighting. The "National Redoubt" of the Nazis in the Alps remained a very real threat to us. We wondered if the Third Army might be ordered to storm it; we hoped not. While we were in Trefelstein a 35-piece German band marched in to surrender in a body to "A" battery—musical instruments and all. We had our aid station in a nice five-room apartment (including bath!) in a small apartment house, so we enjoyed our stay there.

One day while we were there we picked up an American soldier and a British Tommy who had recently escaped from German prison camps. The American had been a prisoner for 10 months, but the Tommy had been a prisoner for five years. He had been captured just before Dunkerque. Both men said all that had kept them alive had been the Red Cross prisoner-of-war packages.

On April 30 we moved to a new location just outside of Waldmünchen, Germany, and on May 1 we moved again, this time across the border to Haselbach, Czecho-Slovakia. It was in this position that our battalion fired its 150,000th round. The next day, during a freak snowstorm, the Second Infantry Division relieved us, and we pulled back into Germany to Lam and then to Lohberg. There we were in the foothills of the Bavarian Alps, and the mountain scenery was most beautiful. At Lohberg we located our aid station and command post in a pleasant German summer-resort hotel. The next day we moved again, to Tresdorf, Germany. It was while we were there that the Eleventh Panzer Division surrendered to our division. The Eleventh Panzer was one of the crack combat divisions of the German army, although it was not S.S. We had fought them before, and we knew their abilities. Now they were facing us on the Czech border, but they no longer wanted to fight. Their commanding general realized that the war was lost for Germany and that further resistance was useless. Besides, he had lost contact with higher headquarters. On May 3 he communicated with the 90th Division and asked to surrender his force en masse. This was done the next day, the surrender being received by the 357th Infantry. All day long lines of enemy tanks, half-tracks, guns and so forth drove into our lines, loaded with fully armed German soldiers. It all went according to plan, however. The soldiers parked the vehicles in orderly rows, laid down their arms and were marched off to prison camps.

Chapter Fifteen

CZECHO-SLOVAKIA AND THE END OF THE TRAIL

*L*ATE IN THE AFTERNOON OF MAY 4 WE LEARNED that we were to go into action once again. Our mission was to advance into Czecho-Slovakia and to secure a bridgehead for the Fourth Armored Division through a mountain pass. Then the Fourth Armored Division would go through us and start a dash across the Bohemian plains.

The next day we started our long drive to our new location in a cold pouring rain. Peter Wedl, Sergeant Frazior and I, in our open jeep, were soon soaked through, and then for many long hours we shivered in our wet clothes as we drove along in the downpour. All of us kept wondering "How much longer can this miserable war last?"

Hitler was reported dead, the German troops in Italy had surrendered and enemy resistance had ceased in Austria and in northern Germany. In fact, the only Allied army on the Western front still in action was the Third Army. We were facing several hundred thousand German troops in the Czech "pocket," whose commander, an S. S. general, had said he would not surrender. Would they fight to the last or would they quit? If they chose to fight it out, of course we would annihilate them, but many more of us would die in the process, and the thought of death, now that victory was so near, was more unpleasant than ever. About dark we pulled into the battered Czech town of Paseka, where we set up our aid station.

The next day, May 6, we sat in place while the tanks of the Fourth Armored roared past on their way into the interior of Czecho-Slovakia. About 0900 we were electrified by a communication received by our anti-aircraft boys: "Between 1000 and 1400 hours a German transport plane may appear over the division area. Do not fire at it!" Then we knew that peace envoys must be on the way, and speculation was rife.

Late in the afternoon we moved over a terrible, muddy, back-woods road to Unterreichenstein. My jeep and truck almost got stuck several places but they managed to get through. Many vehicles were bogged down. On the way I saw the bodies of two enemy soldiers killed the day before, and I thought of the 10 boys from the 357th Infantry killed in an ambush that morning. Once again I shuddered at the uselessness of blood shed in these closing hours of the war in Europe. Although Unter-reichenstein was a Czech town, we were still in the Sudetenland, where most of the inhabitants were German. It was just like being in Germany. They hung out white flags and greeted us in fear and silence.

Finally it came: the long waited-for news. I was standing in the command post about 10 o'clock on Monday morning, May 7. One of the telephones rang. An officer answered it, and then turned to us and said: "The war is over!" No one cheered. No one fired off his gun. The news was too big for that—too awesome. We simply stood there looking at each other and saying, "The war's over at last!" Then the telephone rang again, and we received the division orders. We were to remain in place, take any Germans prisoner, who came in and not fire unless fired upon.

That afternoon Peter Wedl and I drove to Suscice, a fairly large town about 10 miles away, to locate the division artillery aid station. On the way we passed from the Sudetenland into old Czecho-Slovakia, and it was like going from night to day. Instead of a cold, silent, hostile populace, we found crowds of cheering, flower-throwing, rejoicing people waving Czech flags. What a welcome we got in Suscice! It was like France, only more so. I think every citizen must have been out in the streets cheering us, their liberators, and laughing, waving Czech, American and Russian flags, throwing flowers and so forth. The town was decked out for a great holiday, and many of the women were dressed in their beautiful colorful native costumes. I hated to return to Unterreichenstein.

The next day, May 8, the battalion moved to Schihebetz, a little town in old Czecho-Slovakia, and what a great welcome we received! The people were deliriously happy to see us, and they treated us like honored guests. They had a village ceremony of thanksgiving for their deliverance from the Germans, at which they presented our battalion with a little Czech flag mounted on a little flagpole and base. The town band gave concerts in the public square; they had native dances in the open each evening; and they all did everything they could to make us happy. I had a room in a local house for my aid station, and the family was more than gracious to us. They helped us all they could, baked cakes and cookies for us and cooked chickens for us. I soon came to love the friendly, moral, honest, hardworking Czech people.

For two days we stayed here, basking in the warm spring sunshine and enjoying the friendship of the people. After five months in hostile Germany, it seemed good to be among friends again. Some of the American pilots were flying some captured enemy transport planes westward, and now and then we would see these go by overhead. It was strange to watch the big, black, swastika-marked planes lumber across the sky. While we were there we held an impressive memorial service led by Chaplain Cox for our battalion mates who had given their lives in the war.

Then on May 10 we received some disquieting news. The Fourth Armored, out some distance east by itself, reported thousands of enemy troops moving toward them. Whether these troops were coming in to surrender or to attack no one knew so the 90th was ordered to go help the Fourth Armored in case it was attacked. We moved that afternoon farther into Bohemia, thinking, "Won't it be ironical if we have to fight and die now, after V-E Day!" As it turned out, the Krauts were coming in to surrender, much to our relief.

Our drive that day was between cheering throngs of civilians and through gaily decorated towns. Every village and town had put up victory arches across the roads, bearing welcome signs in

149

English and Russian. Home-made Czech, American and Russian flags were everywhere. We passed one large group of German prisoners, and then on one dusty road we passed a parked column of truck-borne Russian troops. What a thrill it was to see our Russian allies, with their close-cropped heads, smiling faces and cheery waves of greeting! We had fought our way a long distance from Normandy to join forces with them. This particular group had come down from the north to contact us. They were riding in American-built trucks.

We drove on to Kateun, where the battalion stopped and went into position, for the division was setting up a defense against possible attack by the Germans to the east. This alert was over in a day or two, for the Krauts wanted no more fighting and surrendered as fast as they could.

One large group of White Russian troops who had been fighting with the Germans against the Reds tried to surrender to our division. Fearing reprisals against them if they gave up to the Reds, they came in to us; but we had orders not to receive the surrender of such troops, so our men simply disarmed them, turned them around and sent them back east to be taken by the Red Russians. I watched them go by, back toward the Reds, as beaten and dejected a group as I have ever seen. I felt a little sorry for them as they rode by on starved, bony horses or on decrepit wagons or walked slowly down the dusty road. They were thin and hungry; their boots were worn and their uniforms were dirty and torn. I wonder if they were massacred by their Red brethren. The Russians were not very charitable toward any other Russians who had fought with the Germans.

We spent four pleasant days in Kateun, taking it easy and enjoying ourselves. We went swimming in some of the small lakes near by; we sunbathed and we just loafed. The townspeople simply could not do enough for us. The whole countryside was having a continuous carnival, and there were dances every night. We established our aid station in a room in a local house again. The family was extremely friendly and helpful. The Czechs were happy to have the Americans there at last.

One afternoon Lieutenant Mann, Lieutenant Murray and 1 drove to Pilsen, about 40 or 50 miles north of Kateun. We saw hundreds of Russian troops on the way. It was most pleasant to drive along across the pretty, rolling countryside on this beautiful spring day. The Czechs were out cheering as usual, and the Russian soldiers waved friendly greetings to us. In Pilsen we drove around to see the city, again receiving the plaudits of the civilians. On the way back we stopped in a tavern in a small town, and soon were surrounded by a friendly, enthusiastic crowd of Czechs. Some of them could speak a little English, and so we had a lively conversation and had trouble tearing ourselves away; but we got back to the battalion by dark.

Soon it came time for the 90th Division to return to Germany to begin its occupation duties in eastern Bavaria, and on May 14 we regretfully took leave of lovely Czecho-Slovakia. Our "liberation tour" had been short in this friendly country, and before long we were back in cold, hostile Germany.

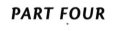

PART FOUR

Chapter Sixteen

OCCUPATION OF GERMANY

*A*LTHOUGH NONE OF US KNEW WHAT THE ultimate plans for the division were, we did know that for a while we were to be occupation troops in eastern Bavaria. The division sector bounded on the east by the western border of Czecho-Slo-vakia extended westward nearly to Nürnberg, and included roughly the territory from Hof in the north to Regensburg in the south. To the 344th Field Artillery Battalion was assigned the *Kreis* (or district) of Burglengenfeld, on the southern edge of the division occupation zone. The battalion set up its headquarters in the little village of Maxhütte, about two miles from Burglengenfeld, (the largest town in the *Kreis*) and about 13 miles from the ancient city of Regensburg on the Danube River.

The battalion convoy rolled into Maxhütte about an hour before sundown on the evening of May 14. Since the housing situation had not yet been worked out, the batteries camped in the open on the first night, just as they had been doing all through the war. The next day we all "moved indoors." Headquarters battery took over the village schoolhouse, a very well-built, two-story building. The first floor was used for the command post and the second for a barracks for the men of the battery. Two of the firing batteries took over a steel mill and the third moved into an abandoned storehouse. The village "Casino" was taken over for the officers' quarters, and for my aid station I appropriated a large room in the attractive home of the more prosperous of the town's two physicians. Later, after things became better organized, I moved my dispensary into a room in the schoolhouse, next to the command post.

For some time the battalion was busily engaged in getting things organized. There were so many things to do, such as getting all our men comfortably settled, deposing the local Nazi *Bürgermeister* and finding a non-Nazi to put in his place, establishing guard posts, getting road patrols started, studying the local economic situation, regulating the great numbers of wandering displaced persons (foreigners from all over Europe), screening and checking the hundreds of demobilized German soldiers who were dejectedly trudging across the country on the way home and so forth.

The two most pressing problems were presented by the displaced persons and the demobilized soldiers. All over Germany were these millions of foreign slaves, whom the "master race" had brought in to work in the fields and factories. Now they were free, but did not know where to go or what to do. First they were gathered into nationality groups, and then as fast as transportation could be arranged they were taken to large collecting points set up by the Army. From there they were sent home. Some of the displaced persons posed a special problem. These were the ones who feared the Russians and whose countries were now under Russian control— the people from Esthonia, Latvia and Lithuania and some of the Poles. They could not go home, under penalty of death. We did the best we could for them. We found them places in which to live and got them food and clothes.

The great hordes of demobilized German soldiers were another problem. Some had been captured in the closing days of the war and had been released, but many others had never been prisoners, and had simply laid down their arms and started home when Germany finally collapsed. At this time they were on the roads by the thousands—dirty, ragged, hungry, demoralized men, wearily walking back toward their homes.

As they entered our *Kreis* they were all checked. If they had been previously checked by American forces and given "clearance papers" they were permitted to go on, but if they had no such papers they were detained for screening. If they proved to be ordinary

Wehrmacht soldiers they were given papers and sent on their way, but if they were found to be S.S. men or war criminals they were arrested and sent to higher headquarters.

Obviously, S. S. troops were not fit to be allowed to return to civilian life, so they were all picked up and put in camps. Many of them, knowing that because of their deeds of horror they were marked men, threw away their S.S. uniforms and tried to pass themselves off as *Wehrmacht* soldiers. But there was one telltale mark. All S.S. troops had had their blood types tattooed on the inner surface of the left upper arm, and so it was a simple matter to order an S.S. suspect to remove his shirt and to look for this mark. Some recently had had this mark excised or had burned it off with a lighted cigarette, but this left a scar. All those with scars in this location were held for further questioning by some of our intelligence interrogators.

This checking of the defeated soldiers was a tremendous task, for they were wandering across Germany in every direction by the millions. How many passed through our battalion area I do not know, but there were hundreds and hundreds of them. We had no place in which to house them while they were being held for checking, and so they were all gathered together in a grove of trees on the edge of Maxhütte, where they pitched their tents and remained under guard until they were released or sent to higher headquarters. Getting food for them was quite a problem, but we were able to draw rations for them from German army food supplies captured by our army. If their homes were in the American or British zone and they were not S.S. men or war criminals they were permitted to continue hiking home. Since arrangements had not yet been worked out with the Russians, those whose homes were in the Russian zone could not go home, and were sent to Weiden, where the 90th Division operated a huge prisoner-of-war stockade for such troops.

Quite a few of the homeward bound troops were sent to me for medical care. They were a ragged, dirty, weary, dejected bunch. I took care of many of them who had old war wounds, infections, injuries, scabies, lice and the like, and I was astounded at the poor medical care the German soldiers had received from their army.

Degeneration of German medicine under Hitler, with a breakdown in organization and a total lack of supplies toward the end of the war, made their medical care hopelessly inadequate.

Then, too, as utter defeat crushed in on Germany, almost no one was exempted from military service, and so there was many a beaten, weary soldier limping home, either so old or so disabled that he ought never to have been in the army. To judge by the great numbers of soldiers with missing extremities I saw, the German surgeons must have been quick to amputate. All these soldiers whom I treated seemed to be courteous and grateful for my care. As was usually the case with them, they immediately jumped to attention whenever an American officer addressed them.

There was another group of patients whom I treated at this time who aroused my greatest sympathy—those miserable wrecks of humanity who had recently been released from the horrors of the concentration camps. Hardly had we set up our dispensary in Maxhütte, when the ghostly procession began. Some had escaped from the infamous Flossenbürg concentration camp which had been located not far from Maxhütte, some had been overtaken by the onrushing American columns a couple of weeks before, as the S.S. guards attempted to march groups of them away from the advance of our army, and a few had been "farmed out" among local labor groups.

Those who dragged themselves to my dispensary were a pathetic sight—crushed in body and spirit. They were emaciated to a terrible degree from years of slow starvation; many were badly diseased, and all bore scars all over their bodies from frequent beatings and other tortures. They were from all the Nazi-dominated countries of Europe.

Those who were too sick (I found some with far-advanced tuberculosis and other serious diseases) or too exhausted, I sent back to our army hospitals in my ambulance; while those whom I thought I could care for I sent into a German civilian hospital in Burglengenfeld, where I watched over them, aided by two German civilian physicians whom I ordered to give these patients the best possible care.

All these men had been given large amounts of food by their liberating American soldiers, but because of their long period of starvation they could not handle the food. As a result they were vomiting and had severe diarrhea. It was truly pitiful to see these emaciated creatures surrounded with food for the first time in years, yet unable to eat. Of course, after a couple of weeks in the hospital on a gradually increasing bland diet, such patients were on the road to recovery. Some of them probably made good recoveries from their concentration-camp terrors, but many of them were too broken in body and spirit ever to be of much use as human beings again. That was the Nazi way.

Another of my early duties in Maxhütte was to check on the sanitary situation in our occupation area—the water supply and its purification, sewage disposal, pollution of streams, mosquito control, public-health menaces and the like. Inspection of the water supply was not for the convenience of our men, for as long as I was in Germany we were ordered to drink only the chlorinated water distributed to us from an army engineer water point. I found many stagnant pools in which mosquitoes bred, and several vermin-infested wooden barracks where foreign slave laborers had lived. There some of the men in my medical section got to work "de-bugging" the barracks and putting DDT-treated oil on the stagnant ponds. Groups of German prisoners were detailed to help them in this.

Here I want to mention the tremendous help given to me by Corporal Peter Wedl as an interpreter. Corporal Wedl was my jeep driver through much of the war, and during my stay with the occupation troops he acted as an interpreter. Although I spoke some German, it was not enough to get me very far; but Corporal Wedl spoke such excellent German that I never saw him stop to grope for words. With his help my work was made easier, and I was able to do a better job than I could have done otherwise.

Next I turned my attention to the hospitals in our area. There were five of these at first—four civilian hospitals in Burglengenfeld and one army hospital in Kallmünz about 5 or 6 miles away. The military hospital, which had taken over part of a Catholic orphanage, was soon to be closed out by the U. S. Third Army medical units in charge of all enemy military hospitals, so I had little to do with this one in Kallmünz.

The four civilian hospitals in Burglengenfeld, however, were my concern. Actually, none of them was really a hospital. They were either convalescent homes or makeshift emergency hospitals set up by the German government when things began to go amiss for them during the war. Normally the people of *Kreis* Burglengenfeld had gone to Regensburg for hospitalization, but with the paralyzing of transportation in the Reich by our air corps and the lack of gasoline, emergency hospitals had been set up.

The main "hospital" in Burglengenfeld had been put in the local schoolhouse and was a general hospital with about 150 patients, including 20 victims from concentration camps and about 20 disabled or sick German soldiers. The physician in charge there was Dr. Fritz Schoeps, a competent surgeon from Breslau, who had fled westward from the Russians. His assistant was a woman, Dr. Pleotzki, also from Breslau. These two did all the work with the help of a fair number of nurses. For a while I had to put up with an arrogant German army dental corps captain, who was looking after the soldiers in the hospital, but I soon got rid of this obnoxious person.

Another "hospital" was more exactly a nursing home, run by Catholic sisters. There were about 20 patients there, mostly with chronic diseases, although occasionally a patient with an acute illness would be admitted.

A third hospital contained a large group of 60 or more war orphans who had chronic diseases such as rheumatic fever and tuberculosis, or who had severe disabling injuries or burns sustained in our bombing of German towns. I hated to see these mangled kids, but that's what war does. The physician in charge there was a woman, Dr. Berndt.

The fourth hospital was a children's contagious-disease hospital; it cared for about 15 children with scarlet fever, measles and typhoid fever. A little later we transferred all the less ill or injured orphans to the orphanage at Kallmünz after the army hospital left, and combined the two children's hospitals into one, with Dr. Berndt in charge.

Of course, all the hospitals were pitifully low on supplies. They were trying to work with almost nothing. Immediately I began trying to get more medical supplies for them from German army medical supply dumps captured by our army, and in this I was quite successful. Our army did a good job distributing badly needed medical supplies to civilian hospitals from these captured dumps.

Lack of food was another serious problem among the hospitals. Few, if any, Germans had enough to eat, and the hospitals were even worse off, for the patients were getting only 850 calories a day—not enough for maintenance, without considering convalescence. By dint of hard work and requisitioning captured army food, I got this pushed up to over 1200 calories. For the 22 ex-concentration camp victims I had in the largest Burglengenfeld hospital, I got extra U.S. Army food from our battalion cooks. The cereals, canned foods, powdered milk and so forth I could get for them was much better for their disordered stomachs than the black bread and potatoes in the German diet. At last these poor fellows were eating properly.

The extra food rations I got for the hospitals I ordered to be distributed evenly among the patients, but this did not please the army dentist. He complained to me that the German soldiers in the hospital should get all the extra rations and the civilians should get along as best they could. With great pleasure I told him that for too long the military had dominated Germany and that the dumb submission of civilians to the whims of soldiers should end. I told him that a soldier was no better than a civilian, as far as I was concerned, and that from now on they would all share alike. After that he was silent.

Dr. Schoeps at the largest Burglengenfeld hospital seemed to be a competent man. He cared for all the patients in the hospital—surgical, medical, obstetrical, gynecological and so forth, and was quite busy. Of course, he was terribly handicapped by lack of supplies. He did not even have any anesthetic agents until I got some for him. I followed the condition of the 22 ex-inmates of concentration camps in the hospital closely to be sure they received good care, and of course they did.

Dr. Berndt, who ran the contagious-disease hospital, was married to a physician in the S.S. I later heard that after I had left Germany she was arrested for previous S.S. connections which she had had. She did a fairly good job of running the hospital for me, and was always quite co-operative. She continually wanted Peter Wedl and me to drop in to visit and drink *Ersatz* coffee, but even had we wanted to we could not because of the Army nonfraternization policy with Germans.

There were several other civilians with whom I had business dealings and who were quite co-operative. Herr Seitz had charge of the food distribution for our section of this *Kreis*, a difficult and thankless job. He and I worked long over diets and calories, and I was able to help him obtain more rations for the area. Another man, the public-health official for the *Kreis*, was a most able physician, and I was sorry when he went to Regensburg to take over a larger district.

Burglengenfeld and Maxhütte had not suffered directly from war damage. They had never been bombed, although there was a steel mill in Maxhütte which would have made a good target. Toward the end of the war many smaller towns, in addition to the cities, had been blasted by our bombers. Regensburg to the south had been heavily hit. Many sections of the city were in ruins, and the factory area and airfield were a shambles. All the bridges across the Danube had been blown by retreating S.S. troops during the last weeks of the war. This was a futile and stupid gesture, for although it delayed the progress of our army hardly at all, it denied the Germans the use of bridges across the river after the war ended, thus greatly hindering their reconstruction efforts. Shortly before the S.S. troops fled from Regensburg to escape from the slashing American columns, they hanged two Roman Catholic priests who had suggested that further bloodshed should cease, since the war was obviously lost.

Schwandorf, a town about 8 or 10 miles to the north of and not much larger than Burglengenfeld, had suffered badly from one bombing. During most of the war the people of Schwandorf had watched great fleets of American bombers pass overhead on the way to bomb some other target. At first they ran for air-raid shelters every time the planes came, but since no bombs ever fell on them, they soon stopped doing this. Then, in the early hours before dawn one morning, a few weeks before the end of the war, a fleet of bombers roared over again; but this time bombs fell on the Schwandorf railyards. The attack lasted 20 minutes, but in that time the railyards and one third of the town were destroyed, and 4,000 people were buried in the wreckage of their homes. A German army hospital train which had pulled into the railyards just before the planes came was demolished.

I had many business trips to make to the division artillery headquarters north of Schwandorf and to an American Army evacuation hospital in Regensburg. The main north and south highway over which I travelled in my jeep was clogged with refugee civilians and demobilized German soldiers. It was ludicrous to see the ragged, dejected members of the once-proud and mighty *Wehrmacht* plodding wearily along, and yet it was also pathetic. They straggled up and down the roads singly or in groups of twos or threes by the thousands—dirty, hungry and bedraggled—carrying their few possessions on their backs or dragging them along behind in rickety little carts. Scattered among the soldiers here and there were women members of the army, also walking the many miles home, and now and then a few civilian refugees. Food was very scarce among them.

One day in May, just after Peter Wedl and I had left Schwandorf in our jeep on the way back to Maxhütte, I suddenly saw a body lying on the side of the road. I had been so used to seeing corpses scattered over the landscape during the war that for an instant I felt no surprise. Then with a start I realized that the fighting was over, and that something was wrong. We halted the jeep, jumped out, and found a young woman lying unconscious beside the road. She was a rather nice-looking girl, although she was dirty; her hair was tangled and her knees and arms were scraped and bleeding from her fall. Her pulse was fast and weak and the respirations were rapid and shallow. Apparently she had collapsed from exhaustion, hunger and heat.

We lifted her into the jeep, and soon she became conscious again. While we drove to Burglengenfeld she told us her story. She was now 22 years old and had always lived in Berlin. Seven years before, when she was 15, she had been "selected" by the S.S. organization to be an "S.S. woman." After going to several camps where she was indoctrinated with the proper S.S. and Nazi ideology, she was sent to an S.S. barracks in Berlin. There she was to live with the men—sew and cook for them, sleep with them and in general keep them happy. The more illegitimate children she would bear, the greater glory to the *Führer*. (She said she had had no children.)

Her mother left Berlin during the war and came to Schwandorf, and her father was killed in the bombing. About four weeks before, during the last chaotic days in Berlin, she had left the city and started out on foot to try to find her mother. When she reached Schwandorf she found that her mother had left there and gone to Regensburg, and so she set out for this city to the south. She had eaten very little recently and nothing at all for two days, and before she had gone far from Schwandorf she collapsed. I took her to the Burglengenfeld hospital, where she remained two days until she recovered enough to continue her journey. Germany was full of such broken lives, shattered homes and tragedy.

Regensburg had numerous large hospitals, both military and civilian, many of which were in school buildings or other public buildings, for the casualties from the war had long since filled the established hospitals to overflowing. I made quite a few trips to these hospitals to arrange for the admission of seriously ill German soldiers to the military hospitals and the admission of civilians from *Kreis* Burglengenfeld to the civilian hospitals for care they could not get in the local hospital.

I did not want to become involved in direct medical care of civilians in the occupation area, but I soon found myself nearly swamped in spite of my wishes. I simply could not turn away the sad parade of suffering humanity who came to me for help. In the first place the local physicians were poorly trained and quite inadequate, and had no medical supplies anyway (although later I gave them medical sundries from captured supplies).

I saw all sorts of infections of the skin, much diarrhea, many malnourished children, dehydrated and dying babies, ex-soldiers with poorly treated, draining old osteomyelitis, women with serious menstrual difficulties, breast abscesses, contagious diseases, fractures, bad lacerations, extensive carbuncles and so forth. "Cradle cap" among babies was rampant. This and the other diseases of the skin were due in large part to the fact that since there was no longer any soap in Europe, no one ever really got clean.

I was especially watchful for contagious diseases. One night about 10 o'clock I was asked to see a woman in Maxhütte who was thought to be choking to death. When I reached the house in which she was staying I found a young woman critically ill with diphtheria. She was not a native of Bavaria, but was a refugee from Silesia. Just before the Russians overran eastern Germany she fled westward with her two small children, aged 3 years and 9 months. When she had reached Maxhütte, a local family (complete strangers to her), had taken pity on this weary wanderer and taken her in. She had lost her home and all her belongings, and she had no idea where her husband, a captain in the German army, might be. Now she had diphtheria, and I was afraid her children would get it too. I took her to the contagious-disease hospital in Burglengenfeld, where she died a week or so later. The two children never contracted the disease, but now the local family with whom they were staying had two motherless children to care for indefinitely.

I saw several civilians with typhus. Every time one of these popped up we sent the patient to the hospital and "de-loused" his home and his family with DDT. Some of the victims of typhus recovered, but several, including a small boy, died.

One evening while a group of German women and children were talking together by a country roadside, another small boy wandered up carrying an interesting-looking plaything he had picked up in a field—an unexploded mortar shell. Boy-like, he banged it against a fence post, and it went off with a roar. When the smoke cleared away, one woman and one boy lay mangled and dead, another woman was practically eviscerated, one arm of the boy who had held the shell was shattered, and the other people were less seriously hurt. I gave first aid to the partially eviscerated woman (who later died) and to the little boy. We took them to the Burglengenfeld hospital, where the boy's right arm was amputated at the shoulder. He was in shock, and so, although we were not supposed to give our medical supplies to enemy civilians, I gave Dr. Schoeps a pint of Red Cross blood plasma for the little fellow. I felt sure that the American who had donated this plasma would not deny it to a critically injured boy. He later made a good recovery from this disastrous incident with such a terrible "toy."

Another patient I cared for was a 15-year-old boy in Maxhütte with rheumatic heart disease and severe cardiac failure. He could get no medicine at all, and was miserable from his fluid-filled lungs, his swollen legs and abdomen, his extreme breathlessness, and his racing heart. I was able to keep him much more comfortable with digitalis, aminophyllin, and diuretics, and, although he died a couple of months later, his family were grateful to me beyond words.

I took care of many, many other ill and injured Germans. When it became a nuisance having so many civilians tramping in and out of my dispensary next to the command post all day, I secured a room in a near-by former tavern. There I saw ill civilians every day from 4 to 5 p.m., but I tried to limit these patients to those whom the local physician could not treat. I saw quite a few interesting medical problems there. Gradually, as I was able to secure more supplies for the local physicians, I cut the number of these patients down, until shortly before I left Germany I closed my "civilian office" and acted only in an advisory capacity to the local physicians.

Another duty I had was to examine for venereal disease all girls caught out after curfew. No Germans were permitted to be out between dusk and daylight (except physicians), and violators of this order were arrested, locked up in the Burglengenfeld jail, and tried the next day by a battalion court. All girls thus arrested were examined for venereal disease, and that was my unpleasant job.

A few weeks after arriving in Maxhütte, I had an interesting 10-day trip across Germany on business. Lieutenant Lou Aebischer and I were ordered to proceed to Bad Neuenahr, headquarters of the 15th Army in western Germany, to act as witnesses at a court-martial. We drove there and back in a command car, getting a good look at a large part of Germany. I was impressed by the total destruction of German cities and even large towns. I cannot begin to describe the devastation, but as we drove along we found city after city blasted into a heap of wreckage with hardly one brick standing on another. The shocking sight of a great city reduced to rubble cannot be put into word pictures; once seen, it never can be forgotten.

On the first day of our trip we drove from Maxhütte to Schwandorf, Nürnberg, Neustadt, Würzberg, Aschaffenburg, Darmstadt (which the 90th had taken during the war) and Frankfurt. The country was made up of rolling hills and was interesting and the roads were fair. Of course, all along the way we passed the ravages of war. We stayed all night in the partially intact Hotel Excelsior, operated by the Army for the use of transient officers, amidst the ruins of that once-great city.

The next day we drove on through Wiesbaden to Ehrenbreitstein, which is on the east bank of the Rhine across from Koblenz. We crossed the river on a ferry (all bridges of course had been blown out during the war), drove through the rubble of Koblenz and turned north along the west bank of the Rhine to Andernach, getting a good look at the gorgeous scenery along the river. A short distance north of Andernach we turned west to the headquarters of the 15th Army at Bad Neuenahr, a few miles distant, where we reported in and were given quarters for the night.

The next morning we were informed that the court-martial had been postponed for five days, and we were told to do as we pleased until then. Accordingly, we decided to drive back into France. We drove back to Koblenz and then started down the south bank of the beautiful Moselle toward Trier. It was a fine trip, and I have seldom seen more lovely scenery than along this river. We passed through Brodenbach, where the division had crossed the Moselle the second time, near the end of the war. At Trier we turned south with the Moselle, and soon were in the midst of the Siegfried Line, whose countless pill boxes were now blasted wide open. This whole area was badly torn up, showing the marks of the savage fighting a few months before.

167

Soon we reached familiar territory where we had fought with the division—Perl, Sierk (France), Malling, Cattenom (where the 90th crossed the Moselle in the big drive to take Metz), Basse Ham, and finally Thionville. We were back in France, "among friends" again, and it seemed good. We crossed the Moselle into Thionville and drove through it to Algrange, a little town several miles to the west. This was all familiar territory to us, and in Algrange we got a room in a little hotel Lou knew about. We spent three days there, taking it easy, sight-seeing, driving around Metz and Thionville and so forth. We also spent some time in a fine rest area of the 80th Division in Thionville.

Then we drove north to the city of Luxembourg, where we spent a day. Just by luck we ran into Captain Harold Cason, whom I had known when he was the commander of a rifle company in the 357th Infantry Regiment of the division. He had been severely wounded early in Normandy, and after his recovery he had been put on limited service. Now he was in charge of the military police in the Luxembourg area. Hal got us some fine rooms in the best hotel in the city, showed us around a bit, and that evening drove us over to a little night club in Belgium, just outside of Arlon, about 40 miles or so away. We had a wonderful time talking and dancing with some of the Belgian girls he knew there. The music was furnished by a phonograph playing American dance records.

Later that day we left Luxembourg and drove back to Bad Neuenahr through Koblenz. The next morning the court-martial was held, and that afternoon, after Lou and I had given our testimony, we started on back to the battalion. First we drove north a few miles to the nearest army pontoon bridge across the Rhine, which was at Remagen. There we saw the remains of that famous and historic Ludendorff bridge, which the First Army had captured intact a few months before. We crossed the river and turned south along its east bank toward Frankfurt, where we spent the night in the Hotel Excelsior again. The next morning we got onto the main north-south *Autobahn* along the east side of the Rhine, and drove south through Mannheim, Heidelberg and Karlsruhe. Then we turned east on the *Autobahn* past Stuttgart and Ulm to Munich. There we turned north to Regensburg,

Burglengenfeld and Maxhütte. We were back again after a most interesting trip. The highways were full of convoys of service troops heading back toward France and embarkation to the Pacific Theater. In spite of my longing to get back home, I was glad to be with occupation troops in Germany rather than with those on the way to the C.B.I.

When I returned from this trip, I found plenty of work to be done, so I was quite busy for some time. It was about that time that the venereal-disease problem began to get serious. During the fighting, venereal diseases among our men had been minimal, but soon after we settled down for occupation duties they skyrocketed. Although the Army vigorously ordered the soldiers not to associate with Germans, venereal diseases continued to increase. The nonfraternization policy worked quite well socially, but not sexually. Many factors contributed to this—the lower Continental moral standards, the chaos and broken homes of the war, the degrading teachings of the Nazis, the many homeless and wandering girls and so forth. Then, too, German women were "man-starved." For years most of the young men had been away at war, and now were either dead or prisoners. Women far outnumbered the men, and what men there were, were over sixty or were under sixteen or were war cripples. As a result, the American soldier could pick almost any woman he wanted. Most of the girls welcomed their new "lovers" for the companionship, but the food, soap, cigarettes, candy and so forth liberally contributed by the boys were most welcome in destitute Germany. Then there were the vagabond girls who loitered along the highways, some even carrying blankets, and who would walk into the woods arm in arm with any G.I. who was interested. Their price was a cigarette, a stick of chewing gum, a piece of chocolate or perhaps nothing. This great moral debauch was sad to see. To me the saddest part was the promiscuity of women with children, who had once been good wives and mothers but whose husbands were now dead or missing; and that of young girls from homes which had once been good, and who in normal times would have been going to school and growing into decent women. Among the German women many surely remained virtuous, but many, also, did not.

As would be expected, venereal diseases, especially gonorrhea, were prevalent among the civilians, and soon the incidence of gonorrhea reached major proportions among our men. Every time I diagnosed an instance, my duty was to learn the names of the female contacts, have them picked up and examine them. If I found the girls to be infected, I had to treat them until they were cured. Soon I had so many diseased girls on my list that I found it difficult to supervise their treatment and carry on my other duties, too, so I opened a venereal-disease ward in the main Burglengenfeld Hospital. There I sent all civilian patients with venereal disease for Dr. Schoeps to look after. Some of the soldiers who contracted gonorrhea I treated in the aid station with penicillin and some I evacuated to the clearing station. In spite of the Army discouragement of fraternization, the numerous prophylactic stations we set up, the frequent medical talks to the men and the many prophylactic kits issued, venereal disease remained a serious problem. It was tragic to behold.

Soon, too, illegitimate pregnancies began to appear frequently. Quite often such girls would come to me asking me to do an abortion, since the fathers of the unborn children were American soldiers. Of course, I absolutely refused to do this and steered as clear of the miserable mess as I possibly could.

The Army attempted to keep the men interested in other matters. Every few nights we had a movie in the battalion area, and frequently U.S.O. shows were put on for us. We built athletic fields and formed a softball league. About 40 riding horses were procured from enemy troops who had surrendered to us, and were kept in a battalion stable for the use of all the men. I loved to ride, and spent about an hour each evening and a couple of hours on week ends riding across the countryside. A fairly good post exchange was set up for us. A fine dock and several diving boards were built at the local swimming pool (or small natural lake) for our men. In addition, German buildings and homes were taken over for the men, to give them all adequate quarters.

The general health of the men was good except for the too-frequent gonorrhea and the great amount of diarrhea. All during our stay in Germany as occupation troops, we were plagued with severe, recurrent diarrhea. It was sporadic and unpredictable, and no one ever found the cause, so far as I know. It did not seem to be carried in the food or water. The diarrhea varied from very slight to extreme, with high fever, chills, vomiting and excruciating abdominal cramps. At times it reached epidemic proportions, and was a serious problem to military operations during the war. Many men were incapacitated by this disease. It seemed to confer either no immunity or a very short immunity, and men were struck by it again and again. I myself was a frequent victim, so I can testify to its severity and persistent recurrence. Since we were immunized against tetanus, typhoid fever and typhus, these diseases gave us no trouble.

All the men and officers were given a turn for a trip to Paris, and my time came on June 18. I decided to try to "hitch hike" a ride in an Army Air Corps transport to Paris and back, instead of going along with the division convoy which spent three hard, dirty, rough days each way in rough-riding Army trucks and bumpy trains. On the morning of June 18 Captain Davis, the battalion surgeon of the 915th Field Artillery of the division, and I got two of our artillery cub pilots to fly us in a couple of cub planes to a big Army air field near Nürnberg (about 50 miles away). After we landed there we ate lunch at the field mess and then located a pilot who was leaving soon to fly his C-47 to Paris. Transport planes were loading and taking off by the dozens, and it was easy to find one going to Paris. The pilot with whom we talked said he'd be glad to take us along as passengers, so soon we were in the air, bound for Paris.

It was interesting to look down on the territory across which we had fought so bitterly, and it seemed strange that we were flying in a few hours over a distance which it had taken us many months to traverse "the hard way." Many memories crowded to my mind as I looked down on the Rhine River, Metz and the Moselle River. About 1600 hours we landed at an Army field outside Paris, got out of the plane and into a truck, and were driven into the city. There we located the Red Cross headquarters, signed in for a "three-day pass," and were given rooms in one of the better hotels, which had been taken over by the Red Cross for the use of

American troops on pass. We were sent to the Hotel Ambassador, where we were each given a luxurious single room with private bath.

Then, for the next six days we really saw Paris—the Arc de Triomphe, Eiffel Tower, Versailles, Trocadéro, Notre Dame, Place des Invalides, Napoléon's tomb, the Louvre, the Folies-Bergère, the Opéra-Comique, the Rue Pigalle, the Bal Tabarin night club, the Montmartre section, the Paris Opéra and on and on. We had a wonderful time. Paris is indeed one of the world's most beautiful cities, and also a very wicked one. Pretty girls could be picked up almost at will if one so desired, and after dark a soldier could not walk a block in the downtown or night-club sections without being accosted by several streetwalkers. It was a "wide open" city, all right.

Since we had flown to Paris, we were able to spend six days there instead of the usual three. However, we had to find lodging elsewhere for the last three nights, for we were given rooms at the Red Cross hotel for only three days and nights. Accordingly, after looking around for a long time, we finally found a room in a little brokendown hotel. The bill for three nights for Captain Davis and me was a total of seven packs of cigarettes.

At last it was time for us to return to Germany. We took a bus to one of the air fields, "hitched" a ride on a plane to Nürnberg, spent the night in the transient officers' quarters, and the next morning were picked up by our cub pilots and flown back to our area. It certainly had been a great vacation for me.

My return, however, was a sad one, for when I got back I found a cable waiting for me telling me of the sudden death of my father, of coronary occlusion. It was a heavy blow to me.

There was much work to be done in our area, and I was kept very busy. Early in July several thousand "displaced persons" moved into *Kreis* Burglengenfeld, most of whom were Latvians. Lithuanians and Estonians. This group of Baltic states people, who had fled in terror from the Russian advance into their home-land, had been in the vicinity of Leipzig and Chemnitz when the war ended. This territory our troops were now turning over to the Russians, and so these people were getting out, too. The Russians hated them, so they must not stay there. Some of them were sent to our area. Men, women and children rode for three days from Leipzig to Schwandorf packed in and on top of old, dirty, rickety box cars. At Schwandorf, trucks from our battalion picked them up and brought them to our area, where they were distributed to all the towns for housing. The *Bürgermeister* of each little town and hamlet was simply told to find room for a certain number of displaced persons who were being sent to his village. This was quite a task, for in war-torn Germany what buildings were left standing were filled to capacity with refugees, and any kind of rooms were at a premium.

The Army authorities were worried about the spread of diseases among these people, so I was ordered to set up some sort of a system whereby all displaced persons in our area could be given a physical examination once every two weeks. When I learned that there were two Latvian physicians and three Estonian nurses in this vicinity, I decided to let them do this work. However, before they could begin, I had a great deal of organization and ground work to do. My first job was to locate the physicians and nurses and enlist their aid.

The nurses I found in the village of Pirkensee, a few miles from Maxhütte, living in an old schoolhouse. Their only possessions were packed in some battered suitcases, but somehow they managed to have some clean uniforms. They said they would be most happy to help.

I had more trouble finding the two physicians. It was a rainy day when we started out to look up the physicians, and Peter and I slipped and slid in the jeep as we drove over the muddy back roads from village to village. At last we found one of the physicians, with his wife and small son, living in a leaky barn along with a group of his fellow countrymen. The common "bedroom" for the entire group was the haymow. Rain dripped down from cracks in the roof, and it was a forlorn group of people who huddled there in the damp, clammy air. The physcian had a few suitcases in which he and his wife had packed what few things they had been able to take of their lifetime's possessions when they had fled from their home. He seemed very happy that I wanted to use his professional services. After a good bit more hunting, I found the other physician, and my "team" was complete.

Next I had to find adequate living quarters for them in a centrally located place. In Burglengenfeld I found a rather nice German home which was not fully occupied, so I merely told the owners that we were taking over part of it. To the nurses we gave two rooms upstairs, to the married physician two other upstairs rooms and to the single physician a room downstairs.

I decided to have my medical team make the rounds of the *Kreis*, rather than to have the displaced persons make long trips to Burglengenfeld from the outlying villages. For this I needed a car for them. The Army had confiscated all civilian cars and had them in a motor pool at Schwandorf, from where they were issued to authorized civilians. After much red tape we finally got one for the use of our medical team. I assigned one of my men to drive the car wherever needed. Since he and one of the physicians both spoke Polish, they were able to communicate with each other. (All my professional helpers spoke German, Estonian, Latvian, Russian and a few words of English, and, as I said, one physician spoke Polish.) The car we used looked fairly good, but, like most European motor vehicles, it did not run well, broke down frequently, and was not easily repaired with the very few parts then available in that wretched part of Europe.

My next task was to find just where all the displaced persons in the *Kreis* had been placed and to look over their health and the sanitary arrangements. Conditions were none too good, but were about as much as could be expected in war-torn Germany. People were crowded into abandoned schoolhouses, old, drafty public buildings, dilapidated barracks and even in barns. As many at 15 or 20 men, women and children often lived and slept in a single large room in a brokendown public building. Privacy was at a minimum, and cooking and sanitation facilities were inadequate. Of course, they had few clothes, shoes, or other personal belongings. They were truly tragic, pitiful people.

As I got to know these Baltic states people I came to like and respect them. They were in general honest, educated, hard-working democratic people, who had great admiration for the United

States and all things American. I had many long talks with them, and learned much about them and their countries. They had been oppressed by both the German and the Russian conquerors. Of the two, German domination was bitter but Russian oppression was intolerable. Consequently, just before the Russian forces retook their lands in the great offensive in the east, most of the citizens fled westward with the Germans. Now they had no country, no homes, and few possessions. Many families were scattered and broken. Probably their countries were gone forever. Most of them longed to get to fabled America, but all they asked was entrance into some safe haven where they could start again to rebuild a good society. Canada and Australia were often mentioned as possible places. I am confident that they will benefit any country which takes them in, and will make fine, loyal, upright, productive citizens.

Next I selected 8 or 10 villages scattered throughout the *Kreis* to which all the displaced persons near them were to come at regular intervals for physical examination by the medical team. Peter and I visited these towns and ordered the *Bürgermeisters* to furnish us with rooms for the examinations and to notify all displaced persons in their areas when to appear.

It was up to me to furnish the team with medical supplies and equipment, and this was quite a task. However, I managed to get a fair supply for them from captured enemy medical dumps.

My troubles did not stop when my medical team finally got started. It seemed as though I always had a dozen or so problems to iron out, some big but most little. From then until I left Germany, this team made complete rounds of the *Kreis* once every 2 weeks, examining the displaced persons. It really "kept me hopping" to keep the system running smoothly.

When the Fourth of July rolled around we had a holiday. In the morning we had a battalion review, during which the guns of our batteries fired 48 rounds of red, white and blue smoke shells. The afternoon was devoted to sports.

To help us with the work in our area, about 100 or more of the prisoners of war who could not return to the Russian zone were sent to us from the division stockade at Weiden. They were quartered in a run-down prison camp which had previously held foreign slave laborers, and were used to do the manual labor around our area. Because many of them were in poor physical condition, I was asked to pass on their ability to work.

Accordingly, one morning I visited the camp to check over the prisoners. They were all sitting in a large barracks, but at the cry of *"Achtung!"* when I entered the room, they all sprang to rigid attention. I had them pass before me, and briefly inspected each man, classifying each for the type of work he could do. I found many of them unfit for heavy labor. Inguinal hernias, stiff knees, injured legs, old age and bad shoulders were some of the disabilities. They were really a poor-looking lot, and for many of them I ordered light work only.

Late in July the Third Army decided to stage a series of raids to check on underground activities, hidden arms, black-market activities and illegal travel. Each tactical unit was ordered to pick out a town in its area and raid it on a certain date. Our commanding officer and his staff chose Kallmünz for our "target." Kallmünz was a small, dirty, crowded, rambling village some distance from our command post at Maxhütte. It was down in a valley along the Nahe River, and we had received reports of some troublemakers there. Once or twice after dark there had been shots fired in Kallmünz. Our plans were carefully and secretly laid. One morning the battalion arose before daylight, boarded trucks and descended on Kallmünz from all sides just as the sun came up. The men got everyone out of bed, sent them all outside of town into a big field, checked everyone's papers, and searched every house from top to bottom. Two suspicious men were sent to headquarters for questioning and a small amount of black-market goods was confiscated, but nothing really exciting occurred. After the search, the startled, sleepy-eyed, strangely dressed townspeople filed back to their homes.

Because the war was still on, we were ordered to continue our training, since we might still be sent to the Pacific Theater (a thought we all dreaded). Every now and then our firing batteries fired their guns on a range which had been laid out. We were also preparing for a field problem with the infantry of several weeks' duration late in September. We hated the prospect of moving out into the field and again sleeping on wet ground during the chilly September nights, but orders were orders. Then August came, and the end of the war with Japan. We waited anxiously for the final word during those suspense-filled days preceding V-J Day, and were filled with joy and thanksgiving when the surrender took place. We were also very pleased when all training programs were immediately cancelled, including the hated field problem.

And so the summer dragged by. All of us longed to get home, especially now that the war was over. We knew, of course, what a tremendous task it would be to get us all home, so we did not expect to get back very soon. "Discharge Points" were the main topic of conversation. Before V-J Day, my 78 points were not enough to get me home, but with the recounting after V-J Day, I had just enough—the 85-point minimum. I lived in hopes of a speedy return home, but really never expected to get back soon.

Early in September, Lieutenant Thorpe, Major Swotash and I received permission to take a 6-day motor trip through southern Germany and western Austria. We left on the morning of September 6 in a command car, and what a fine trip that was! The first morning we drove to Munich, which, as we knew, had been destroyed in the bombings. We ate lunch at an officers' mess, and in the afternoon drove up to see the Dachau concentration camp, a few miles northwest of Munich. Part of it was now used to confine a large group of S.S. prisoners, but the rest was open to Allied soldiers for inspection.

The camp was a huge affair, surrounded by two high barbed-wire fences (the outer one of which was electrified), a wide moat, and numerous machine-gun emplacements. The barracks which had housed the prisoners were of wood, but the main buildings were all stone. Outside the camp were many lovely stone homes where the brutal S.S. guards had lived in luxury. It was hard to realize that in this infamous camp thousands of suffering men had lived tortured lives and died in agony.

A young Pole who had spent over a year here as a prisoner acted as our guide. We saw the long rows of kennels where the guards had kept their vicious police dogs, which were used as watchdogs.

At night every S.S. guard who patrolled the grounds had a police dog with him. Not infrequently the guards set dogs on helpless prisoners just for a little "sport." We saw the place near the crematory where the Germans had lined up a large number of high-ranking captured Russian officers. As they had stood there S.S. men had walked along behind them, shooting each one in the back of the head.

Then we saw the gassing chamber. This was a room about 30 feet square with a low ceiling, two doors on opposite sides of the room, and on three of the walls a single, small window filled with solid, unbreakable glass. In the ceiling were dummy shower heads, in even rows. The victims were taken first into an adjoining room where they were ordered to strip off all their clothes. Then they were told that they were to be given a shower, and were herded into the chamber. After all were inside, both doors were locked, and lethal gas instead of water was turned on. When S.S. guards, peering through the three little windows, reported that all signs of life in the enclosed mass of humanity had gone, the gas was shut off, air was run in, the doors were opened, and the corpses were hauled to the nearby crematory.

Thousands of men, women and children had been exterminated here. Our guide said that after the abortive Munich beer-hall attempt on Hitler's life in July of 1944, the gas chamber had run continuously for many days. Whole families had been gassed together. Many German officials and army officers, who were suspected of being in on the plot, were arrested, along with their wives and children, and all were executed in the chamber.

From there we walked next door to the crematory. It was a large, high-ceilinged building in which were three huge cremating furnaces. The room was neat and clean, the floor was scrubbed and the walls were whitewashed; but all around the room to a height of about 3 feet above the floor the walls were splashed with old, dark blood, where the corpses had been piled high, awaiting cremation. From the ceilings wooden frames hung down in front of the furnaces. Our guide said the Nazis sometimes suspended prisoners by their arms in front of the furnace doors in an effort to extract information from them. The searing heat of the flames close by, the sight of the bodies of fellow prisoners being tossed into the fire and the added fiendish tortures of the guards were good "tongue-looseners." If the victims finally died without revealing what was sought, they were cut down and added to the cremation pile; if they finally "broke" and told what was wanted, they were immediately cast into the furnace, still living, with about as much concern on the part of the guards as a baker filling his oven.

In the crematory basement were hundreds of large boxes and small urns filled with the charred bones of cremated prisoners. The ashes of the victims were all raked out in a pile together and then many urns, looking like flowerpots, were filled with them. Then the Nazis notified the families concerned that so and so had died, and that for a sum of money ($100, I believe) they could have his ashes. If the grieving family paid, they received an urn containing everyone's ashes but their loved one's. The "unbought" ashes were used to fertilize gardens in the guards' homes.

We left the depressing sights of Dachau and returned to Munich, where we turned south and soon were in the beautiful Bavarian Alps. About 1800 hours we reached the quaint little village of Oberammergau, noted for the famous Passion Play. We located a caretaker of the Passion Play Theater who agreed to show us through (for which we paid him a couple of K rations). Oberammergau had not been touched by the war, and hence everything was intact. The Passion Play Theater is a huge, dome-shaped steel building with one end open. At this open end is a stage, exposed to the weather, and from the stage row after row of seats rise toward the back of the theater, one above the other. Behind the stage are many rooms, in which are stored the costumes and scenery. We saw the costumes for the temple guards, the Roman soldiers and the disciples, the table for the Last Supper, the crosses for the crucifixion, the shields, spears and helmets of the soldiers and the like. It was a most interesting sight. Every ten years, in normal times, the Passion Play is presented once a day all summer long, to great crowds from all over the world. Oberammergau was a Nazi town, however, in spite of its religious history. The caretaker who showed us around was a one-armed German army veteran. Like most people of the town, he had formerly appeared in the Play. He had taken the part of a temple guard.

After that we drove to the tiny town of Linderhof, near one of the two gorgeous palaces built by the mad King Ludwig II of Bavaria. Since it was getting dark we decided to stop for the night and see the palace in the morning. We found a nice Alpine resort hotel and stopped there. Of course, there were no other "guests" there, and the proprietor could do nothing else but take us when we said we were staying for the night. He had no sheets or blankets, but we threw our sleeping bags on the beds in our rooms and slept comfortably.

In the morning we packed up and then walked over a short trail to the near-by "Schloss Linderhof," which was built in 1874 at tremendous cost. Its builder, King Ludwig II, was an insane prince of Bavaria who had erected two unbelievably ornate and expensive palaces, one here and one some distance away on Lake Chiem. Ludwig had been a bachelor and a woman-hater, and he wanted to be alone most of the time. In his lavish dining room he had a sliding panel built into the floor so that the table could be lowered to the room below, filled with food, and then raised again to him. Thus he could eat alone without seeing a human being. He required any servants who had to be in his presence to wear masks.

Schloss Linderhof is a gorgeous palace, set in a beautiful valley. Lovely gardens, marble walls and statues, terraces and fountains rise from the bottom of the valley up the mountain sides on either side of the palace. High on top of the palace is a large statue of Atlas supporting the world on his shoulders. When the visitor goes inside, he is overwhelmed by the succession of magnificent rooms through which he walks. There are beautiful tapestries, inlaid floors, breath-taking paintings on the walls and ceilings, dozens of statues, intricately carved tables and chairs, curtains woven with threads of spun gold and so forth. It was all a beautiful sight, but so heavily ornate as to be almost oppressive.

After leaving Linderhof we drove on south, deeper and deeper into the Alps. Scenes of great beauty passed before our eyes— majestic, snow-capped peaks, sparkling lakes and dense forests.

We stopped a short time in Garmisch and Partenkirchen, the headquarters for winter sports in Germany and the location of the Winter Olympics in 1936. Then we drove on through Mittenwald into Austria to Innsbruck. Since this part of Austria was being occupied by the French, we were stopped at the German-Austrian border by a road block manned by fierce-looking, bearded, dark-skinned, turbaned French Colonial troops. They were under orders to allow no one to pass through, but finally we persuaded them to take us to their officers a mile or so down the road. After a half-hour or so of discussion by the officers in charge, we were permitted to continue our trip.

A short time later we reached beautiful Innsbruck, lying on the Inn River, nestled in an Alpine valley. We saw no American soldiers—only a few French troops and the tricolor, although the French had complete American equipment from uniforms and rifles to jeeps and trucks. After sightseeing a little in Innsbruck we drove on south to the Brenner Pass. There, high up in the Alps, we passed from Austria into Italy. This narrow pass had been the chief German supply line into Italy during the war, and so our air force had blasted it repeatedly. Although the road had been repaired since the end of the war, it was still almost impassable in places. The railroad running beside the road had been left a complete ruin by our bombers. Entire trains lay smashed along the wrecked tracks, blackened and twisted. Thousands of rounds of shells from destroyed ammunition trains lay scattered around. Over much of the area bomb craters seemed to cover every square foot of ground.

We decided to drive down into Italy a short distance, and so we continued on south from the Brenner Pass. Shortly before sundown we came into a beautiful wide, green, fertile valley in which lay the pretty town of Bressanone. We were getting tired and hungry and so when we passed a command post of a battalion of the 88th Division we stopped. The 88th had fought a long, hard war up the rugged Italian countryside, and now was policing the area. This particular battalion was policing the part around Bressanone. The officers were most cordial and invited us to spend the night with them.

We walked around town a bit and then had dinner and spent the evening at the officers' club, which was in a fine villa along a rushing river at the edge of town. The club had been beautifully decorated, and captured German soldiers waited on the tables in fine style. A small band played for dancing, for, since Italy was not a "conquered country," American troops could "fraternize" as much as they wished. Since huge stores of German army liquors had been captured near the place, all sorts of fine, rare drinks flowed like water. It was quite a "setup" for these boys.

The natives around were mostly tall and fair, and not at all like the short, dark Italians farther south. This was because this part of Italy had belonged to Austria before the first World War, but had been given to Italy at the peace conference. Most of the natives were still loyal to Austria and were opposed to Italian rule. Feelings ran high between Italian and Austrian nationalists, and clashes were frequent. The American troops were there to preserve order and prevent a local uprising.

Late that evening we decided to drive several hundred miles south into Italy to see Venice the next day. In the morning we arose before daylight and started out about 0400 hours. All morning we drove through mountainous, interesting country. Mountain houses, quaint native villages, terraced slopes and vineyards made interesting scenery. Although we were on the main road south, it was none too good, and our ride was a bumpy one. Gradually the terrain became less rugged, and soon opened out into broad, fertile plains.

By about 1300 hours we were only 18 miles from Venice, but then our plans went amiss. The command car broke down, but it so happened that a short distance down the road was a British army installation. These fellows were very kind, got out a truck, and towed us to an R.A.F. automobile maintenance shop in the next town. It was a Saturday afternoon and they were not working, but a couple of mechanics volunteered to help us, and after much difficulty had the motor going again by 1600 hours. The water pump had broken, but they patched it up. They had no parts for Dodge trucks, so they could not replace the pump.

About 1700 hours we reached Venice, and what an interesting place it is to see! The city is built on a great many tiny islands in the Adriatic Sea, connected to each other by foot bridges. One cannot drive a vehicle into the city, for there is no automobile bridge to it in the first place and no streets wide enough for cars in the second place. All travel in Venice is on foot or by gondola on the maze of canals. I had thought that probably the ancient and picturesque gondolas had long since disappeared except for a few for tourist attractions, but this was not then the case. At that time gondolas were still the Venetians' chief mode of transportation, and they were speedier than one would imagine. We drove our command car to the outskirts of the city, left it in a large parking garage and rode into Venice proper in a British army motor launch. The British were administering this part of Italy. We docked at one of the main landing places, got out of the launch, and started walking through the narrow, crowded cobblestone streets toward Saint Mark's Square, near which we knew were two hotels for transient Allied officers. What a change this was from the ravaged cities of smashed Germany! There was no war damage in Venice itself (only the oil refineries outside the city had been bombed). Crowds of well-dressed, laughing Italians thronged the streets, and the shops were filled with fine clothes, jewelry and other goods (although most things were very expensive and could not be procured without ration coupons).

Soon we found our billet for the night, one of the best hotels in Venice. We signed in and were given fine rooms. Lieutenant Thorpe and I shared a luxurious double room, with bath, in the front of the hotel. Outside our windows was a balcony overlooking the famous Grand Canal, the "Broadway" of Venice. Next we started on some sight-seeing. We visited Saint Mark's Square, went through Saint Mark's Cathedral, and then walked over to the nearby gondola "stand." There we hired a gondola for an hour's trip and had a most delightful excursion. We leaned back on the cushioned seats and enjoyed the sights as the gondola slipped smoothly and quietly over the canals under the skillful sweep of the gondolier's oar. We floated by the Doges' palace, the Rialto, the Bridge of Sighs and many other interesting and historical landmarks.

Since the people empty their garbage and other refuse out the windows into the canals, the water is not exactly pure, and I would hate to fall in. It surprised me to see that the canals were truly the "streets" of Venice, and that the houses were built right on the water's edge, with the front door opening directly onto the canal.

After dinner we went for a long walk through the maze of narrow streets running across the islands of the city, crossing canal after canal on the little picturesque foot bridges. It was Saturday night, and a gay throng of people were out pleasure seeking. Music was everywhere. Here and there we saw tied up together in a canal a couple of boats loaded with people. Many flickering lanterns lighted the scene, while the people sang beautifully to the accompaniment of accordions and guitars. Passing crowds would stop to listen, and then walk on.

After a while we returned to our hotel, and for a long time I sat on the balcony outside our room watching the scenes on the Grand Canal below. It was a warm, beautiful night, with a low-hanging moon. Dozens of gondolas glided up and down the wide canal, and laughing voices and songs of singing gondoliers floated on the air. Frequently a large boat gaily decorated with swinging colored lanterns would drift by, loaded with singing people. Finally I went indoors and went to sleep under a canopy of mosquito netting, which for obvious reasons enclosed all beds in the hotel.

In the morning after breakfast we took a gondola back to the mainland, loaded into the command car and started north. We had gone only about 50 miles when the water pump began to give trouble again. We knew that the car would never make it back to Bressanone, and so we began to look around for help. A short time later we came to some units of General Anders' Free Polish Army (which had fought in Italy with the British), and there we stopped. Their courtesy and kindness were heart warming. Since they were equipped with American vehicles, they had spare parts and they gave us a brand-new water pump. Two mechanics got up from their Sunday dinner to install it for us, and soon we were on our way again.

We decided to take a different road back to Bressanone, a more or less "back" road, and it was quite a trip. The road was a fairly good gravel thoroughfare, but it ran through wild, rough, sparsely populated Alpine country. Up and down steep grades, around sharp turns, through quaint little isolated villages and past towering mountain peaks we went. It was a most beautiful ride and very interesting, but we were a bit relieved when, early in the evening, we again reached Bressanone.

When we arrived at the command post of the battalion of the 88th Division where we had spent the night previously, we found it bristling with machine guns, rifles and mortars. The officers explained that there had been some trouble over the week end between Italian and Austrian nationalists, and so they were prepared for any emergency. No more came of it, however.

The next morning we started north, back up across the Alps, through the Brenner Pass and back into Austria. At Innsbruck we turned east toward Salzburg. Along the way we turned off on a side road to see an underground aircraft factory built by the Germans. They had enlarged an old mine in a mountainside into a small factory, had run in electricity and had hundreds of machines in it for the manufacture of parts for Heinkel planes. There they were safe from Allied bombings.

Late that afternoon we reached Berchtesgaden, Hitler's mountain retreat. I was quite surprised at the large number of buildings here; it had really been a small village. Near the end of the war it had been heavily bombed by the R.A.F. and later burned by the S.S. troops before they fled. We walked through the ruins of the houses of Hitler, Goering, Bormann, the S.S. men and others. In Hitler's house we saw the place where his famous view window had been. All these houses were connected by tunnels. Then we descended into the deep, underground stronghold, where the Nazis had hoped to hold out. There were long corridors and dozens of rooms—bedrooms, bathrooms, kitchens, storerooms, sitting rooms—some of them partially furnished. Every few hundred feet there was an L-shaped jog in the corridor, and at each turn there was a machine-gun emplacement. From these steel guard posts, S.S. men could protect this underground hideout, and sweep the halls with machine-gun fire.

After leaving Berchtesgaden we drove into near-by Salzburg for the night. The next morning we looked around Salzburg, which is an interesting old Austrian city indeed. One of its most interesting sights is the medieval castle which stands on a high hill. We went all through it with an informative guide.

From Salzburg we drove westward, over a good highway, stopping at the beautiful Lake Chiem. The sparkling blue waters with the snow-capped Alps in the distance made a lovely picture. King Ludwig (the same old fool who had built the magnificent palace at Linderhof) had constructed another palace, even more ornate than Linderhof, on an island in the middle of the lake. We took the little excursion launch from the mainland to the island, called Herren Chiem See, and spent several interesting hours wandering through halls and rooms of unbelievable splendor. One huge, ornate hall was patterned after the famous Hall of Mirrors in Versailles, but to me it far surpassed the beauty of its pattern. This palace of Ludwig was in the same style as that at Linderhof, except even more ornate, larger and on a more grandiose scale.

After returning to the mainland we got back into our command car and started west again, reaching Munich about dinnertime. We had dinner there at the transient officers' mess, and returned once more to Maxhütte at about 2200 hours.

We got back on September 11, and when we did we found that a large number of the higher-point men had been transferred out of the battalion to go home with other divisions returning soon to the States. I lost all but about three of the men from my medical detachment. A few other men were transferred in to me, but we were still far under strength and had trouble carrying on our routine tasks. Among the men transferred out was Peter Wedl, my ace interpreter and helper, and that was a blow. However, I rejoiced that my boys who had served their country so faithfully and so long were at last going home.

Chapter Seventeen

HOME AGAIN

*I*N THE DAYS THAT FOLLOWED, MORE AND MORE men of the battalion started on their way home. The 90th Division was not scheduled to leave until December, but all its high-point men were to go home with other outfits. As a result, our affairs were chaotic as we tried to carry on our duties in the face of the rapidly changing and dwindling personnel. "Going home" was on everyone's lips. Like all the others, I was burning with the desire to get home, yet I was willing cheerfully to obey orders and to stay in Europe as long as I was needed.

So far as my discharge points were concerned, with the recount after V-J Day I had exactly 85, and 85 was that magic number which meant early discharge. Men with 85 points or more were reported to be going home soon, but those who had fewer than this number were "out of luck" for a while, at least. Had I entered the Army three days later than I did, or had V-J Day come three days earlier than it did, I would have had one point less, or 84. I was very lucky in that respect.

As I said before, I was anxious to go home, and I hoped fervently for some miracle to start me on my way; but I honestly felt that it would be many more months before I would see the United States again. On September 13 several of the higher-point medical officers were transferred out of the division to the Twelfth Armored Division in Czecho-Slovakia, which was preparing to go home in a month or so, and how I envied them.

Then on September 17, just 6 days after I returned from the trip to Austria and Italy, the miracle happened! It was about 1400 hours and I was watching a ping-pong tournament in the enlisted men's club, when one of the men said, "Telephone for you, Captain." I walked to the phone, wondering who was hurt or sick.

"Doc," said the voice of Major Spencer, the battalion executive officer, "can you stand a shock? You have orders to fly home at once."

I was too stunned to know what to think. "Major, you're joking!" I said incredulously.

"No, I'm not, Doc," he answered. "You are to be at division headquarters by seven o'clock tonight, so you'd better hurry."

I put down the phone and walked away in a daze. Flying home! It couldn't be true! It couldn't! I was too elated to think clearly. I was simply walking on air. Since division headquarters were two hours' drive away, I would have to leave not later than 1700 hours, and that gave me only 3 hours in which to get ready.

I hurried back to my room, quickly packed the old suitcase I planned to take with me, threw the rest of my belongings in a heap on my bed, and asked Sergeant Lisne, my section sergeant, to pack them in my foot locker for me and ship it home. Then I went to the aid station to bid farewell to my men and to the command post to get my orders. By then it was 1645 hours, and time to leave, so Corporal Hadcock, my driver, brought around our jeep and I took a last look at Maxhütte as we started for division headquarters.

The circumstances surrounding my unexpected trip home were so lucky and coincidental that I think they are worth repeating. To begin with, I flew home on the Green Project. Because of the clamor in Congress to get physicians home soon, the War Department ordered early in September that 6,000 high-point medical officers be flown home within 2 weeks. This was under the "Green Project," which had already flown back many high-point men.

My first good fortune was in having the required 85 points, which I had just barely amassed. The second lucky break was that just 4 days before, the highest-point medical officers had been transferred out of the division. Had they been there when the Green Project orders came through, I would not have been included. A third happy coincidence was that I had taken the trip into Austria and Italy when I did and not a week later as I had once planned, or I would have missed returning home at this time.

Another lucky thing was that the division personnel office was able to slip me in "under the wire" in the following way. Corps headquarters telephoned the 90th division to send five medical officers with 85 points or more on the Green Project. After checking the records the division reported to Corps that they had five doctors with over 85 points and one with an even 85. Could they send all six instead of the requested five? After some deliberation, Corps headquarters approved. Had they refused this request I would of course have been left behind.

But my luck did not stop here. The division personnel office could not establish contact with our battalion to give them my orders, but just as they were about to quit trying, the telephone lines cleared and they got through. They told one of the battalion personnel clerks what they wanted, and asked him to check on my points. By some mistake he reported that I had only 60, so the division office crossed my name off the list. By another coincidence, Major Goodman, the division artillery surgeon, was in the division office at this time, and said he knew I had more than 60 points. They then asked the battalion clerk to recheck the records. He found his mistake and said I had 85, and my name was put back on the list. I did not know all this while it was going on, and I am glad I did not. That saved a lot of wear and tear on my nervous system at a time when I could have least afforded such a psychologic insult.

When I reached division headquarters about 1830 hours, I found the other five medical officers already assembled. I was happy to see that one of them was Jack Gable, my good friend and fellow infantry battalion surgeon. I learned that we were to drive to Munich, about 150 miles to the south, that night and get a plane for Paris in the morning.

After dinner at the division officers' mess (although we were too excited to eat much) Jack, one of the other officers, and I climbed into a command car, and the driver started south. Soon it got dark, but we were on an *Autobahn* leading to Munich, so we could roll along at a good clip. As I sat in the back seat, staring out into the darkness, with the cold night air whipping across my face, I found it hard to believe that I was on my way home. *Home!* Oh, what that word stood for! Was the miserable nightmare of war really only an unpleasant memory? Was it all behind me, and had I somehow lived through it? Was I really leaving the devastation and hunger and misery of Germany? Was I truly going to be back soon to my beloved wife and little son? It was all too good to be true.

About midnight we reached Munich, located the transient officers' quarters, and were assigned bunks in a large wooden barracks. None of us was interested in sleep, but we did get in a few hours in spite of our excitement. Soon after sunrise Jack and I got up, washed, packed our things, ate breakfast, and went over to the near-by air field from which Army transports were leaving every few minutes. After standing in line a long time we reached the dispatcher's window and were assigned to a plane leaving for Paris about noon. Most of the morning Jack and I spent lying on the grass watching the planes come and go and talking over our war experiences, the trip home, our families and our post-war hopes and plans.

At last our turn came; we loaded onto the plane, the C-47 roared down the runway and we left the soil of Germany behind. About three hours later we landed in Paris. We did not know where to go from the airport, but about 15 or 20 of us "Green Project" medical officers took an Army bus into the center of the city. We got off at the Place de l'Opéra, but had no idea where to go from there, and so we stood on a corner, looking very much like a group of wandering sight-seers. Carrying our heavy baggage, we walked several blocks to a couple of offices of different Army units. At last someone was able to tell us where to go, so we hired a rickety old French bus and rattled off through the bewildering maze of the streets and cul-de-sacs of Paris to our final destination.

The headquarters of the Green Project were in an old former department store near the Montmartre section of Paris. Partitions had been built, dividing the huge open floors of the store into many large rooms, into which hundreds of wooden bunks had been put. Sleep was difficult in these barracks, with men coming and going at all hours of the day and night, but no one cared much about sleep. We signed in late Tuesday afternoon, September 18, and were assigned bunks. There were about 1,000 medical officers here, some leaving to fly home and others arriving all the time.

The next morning all of us who had arrived the day before met together and were told what we were to do, among which were such things as getting physical examinations done, having our luggage inspected, and weighing in. Then we were shown a moving picture telling us what to do if the plane was forced down at sea. After getting the above requirements completed, I was free to do as I pleased until my turn came to leave. Since no one knew just when flights would be scheduled, we were advised to check the flight lists on the bulletin board several times a day to be sure we wouldn't miss our turn when it came.

As it turned out, I left early Saturday morning, and so I had 3 days in which to wander around Paris some more. I visited the Louvre, where I saw the original Mona Lisa, Whistler's Mother, Winged Victory and Venus, I strolled along the Champs Elysées; I looked into some of the shops on the Rue de la Paix; and in the evenings I relaxed at some of the pleasant sidewalk cafés.

At last came the news I was waiting for. Late Friday evening my name was included in the list of those who were to leave early Saturday morning. I got everything ready Friday evening and then lay down to try to sleep, but what little sleep I did get was fitful, to say the least. About 0500 hours I arose, dressed, and reported at the bulletin board, where our group was to meet. There were about 25 of us in the group.

After we had all assembled we went outside, got into a bus and started for the airport. It was a beautiful, clear, bright, cool day, and the world seemed very wonderful. In about half an hour we arrived at the airport. How good those big, silver four-engine C-54's looked. After a short wait we drove out to one of the planes, loaded into it and in a few minutes were in the air over Paris, headed for home. Our first stop was to be Lisbon, Portugal, as our route led southwest. The French countryside looked very pretty as it slipped along beneath us. A little later we passed Bordeaux, and soon we were over Spain. I was amazed how poor the land of Spain looked from the air; it seemed to consist of barren hills and dry gullies, with little greenness and only a few small villages.

Five hours after leaving Paris we were over Portugal and soon we saw the pretty city of Lisbon, with its gleaming white buildings, wide palm-lined streets and blue harbor. Our plane circled low over it several times before landing, so we got a good look at it. We made an hour's stop there, and so we walked into the airport terminal while we waited and talked with some of the men from the American military mission stationed here. Since Portugal was neutral in the war, we were not permitted to leave the airport, and armed Portuguese sentries guarded the doors to enforce this ruling Salazar, the dictator of Portugal, was a complete tyrant, we were told, and ruled the country with an iron hand. He controlled every phase of national life and much of private life, too. His fierce oppression of any opposition kept him in power. He was a small-time Hitler or Franco, so we were told.

In about an hour we climbed aboard our plane again, took off and headed westward across the Atlantic for the Azores. It seemed strange to look down on water as far as the eye could see. For a while I sat in the pilots' cockpit, watching the crew operate the ship, and then I simply gazed out into space, watching the beautiful formations of clouds through which we flew. In about 5 hours we were approaching the Azores, and while the plane prepared to land we buckled our seat straps and put on our life jackets (to be used in case the ship overshot the field and plunged into the ocean). We had a two-hour stopover, and hence had time to eat supper at the field canteen, walk around a bit, and talk with some of the personnel stationed there. It was a hot, almost tropical climate and the bare rocks gave little protection from the heat.

It was just getting dark when we took off from the island. Ahead were 10 hours of flying over unbroken ocean before we would reach Newfoundland, the next land. Most of us spread blankets on the floor of the big plane and lay down for a little sleep. I was quite tired, and was able to sleep off and on until we were nearly to Newfoundland. It was still dark (about 0400 hours) when we landed at the Stephensville airport (near Gander), and a blast of cold air hit us as we stepped from the plane. After the tropical warmth of the

Azores the ice and snow of Newfoundland seemed colder than ever. While the plane refueled, we ate breakfast in the canteen, served by Canadian girls, the first English-speaking "natives" I had seen since I left England 15 months before. After breakfast we climbed aboard the plane and took off in a howling snowstorm on the last leg of our journey.

The air was very bumpy for the first hour after we left Newfoundland. The big ship lurched and bucked, and particles of ice rattled on the windows as we swayed through the thick weather. At last we climbed above the storm and the clouds, just as daylight came, and thenceforward all was calm.

About 0800 or 0900 hours the crew told us we had crossed the Canadian border and were looking down on the good old U.S.A. How wonderful it was to see our homeland again after all these weary months! We looked down with reverence on the towns and villages and the cars skimming along the highways. Then the great cities of Portland, Boston, New York, and Philadelphia slid beneath us, and finally we saw the large A.T.C. field at Wilmington, Delaware, come into view. Our faithful ship circled the field, glided in for a landing, and then we set our feet once again on the soil of the United States of America. It was about noon on Sunday, September 23, 18 months to the day since I had left the country.

It took us only a few minutes to be cleared by the customs, and then we were driven to temporary quarters, where we shaved and cleaned up, and were given dinner. My first act after we were "turned loose" was to hunt a telephone to call my wife. I had cabled her before I left Paris, so she knew I was on my way home, but by the time the call went through I was so nervous I could hardly talk. However, I did manage to talk, and how wonderful it was to hear her voice!

After the telephone call I walked over to the camp headquarters to find out how soon I could leave. There I was told that I was scheduled to leave the next morning for Indiantown Gap, near Harrisburg, Pennsylvania, for discharge from the Army. However, the clerk told me that if I wanted to pay my own way to the camp I could leave immediately. That was all I wanted to know. Now that I was so close to seeing my beloved Adrienne again, I would do anything to be with her.

I caught a ride into Wilmington, bought a ticket for Harrisburg, and within a short time was on the train. From Harrisburg, I took a bus to the separation center at Indiantown Gap, which I reached about 2200 hours. As any soldier knows, it is difficult to find one's way around a strange army camp after dark, especially on a Sunday night. After much hunting, however, I located the officers' discharge center, signed in, and then found a bunk for the night.

Early the next morning I began making the rounds of the various places in camp through which officers for discharge had to pass. By midmorning I had completed all I could for several days, and I was informed that I could leave camp if I would agree to be back on the morning of the third day. That was the news for which I had been hoping and longing. I telephoned Adrienne to meet me in Pittsburgh at the Fort Pitt Hotel and caught a bus for the Smoky City.

About 2100 hours I arrived at the Union Bus Terminal, and, in a highy nervous and excited state, I walked over to the nearby Fort Pitt Hotel.

"Yes, Captain," the desk clerk said, "Mrs. McConahey has registered."

A bellboy led me to the room. I tried to appear calm, but inside I was in an uproar and my knees just barely supported me. I tipped the bellboy (how much, I have no idea) and knocked. The door opened, and there stood my Adrienne. In a second she was in my arms, and the long separation was over.

And so ends my narrative. Three days later I returned to Indiantown Gap, completed the separation proceedings, and on September 28, 1945, left there, a civilian once again.

ACKNOWLEDGMENTS

"*WHAT I SAW MUST NEVER HAPPEN AGAIN.*"
I can still hear the urgency in Dr. McConahey's voice as he spoke to a group of Mayo Clinic colleagues and guests in the late 1990s. He was describing the liberation of the Flossenbürg concentration camp, and his theme was the tragedy of a world engulfed by war. The stories he shared took us from landing on the beaches of Normandy, France, to the surrender of Nazi Germany.

I knew Dr. McConahey casually at the time and was aware he had written a book about serving in World War II. But it was that day when I grasped the significance of his experience. I wanted to learn more.

Our paths continued to cross in the years that followed. I was a Mayo Clinic administrator at mid-career. He was a distinguished Emeritus Staff physician. I read his book, *Battalion Surgeon,* which provided the basis of conversations I remember and cherish to this day. Dr. McConahey was willing to talk about the war, but he always diverted attention to those he had served with—"They were the real heroes," he would insist. From reading his memoir and knowing the context of what he described, I could see in Dr. McConahey a kind of heroism to which he would never admit. Under combat conditions, at risk to his own life, he provided care for friends and foes, combatants and civilians. "After all," he would say, "I am a doctor."

The volume of *Battalion Surgeon* that I read was privately published in 1966, followed by two versions of limited quantity. Dr. McConahey's story deserved a much wider readership, and I admit that creating a high-quality, accessible edition became a passion project.

Collaboration is the hallmark of Mayo Clinic. A remarkable band of colleagues united their skills for this good cause. The

80th anniversary of D-Day provided the target for our timeline. It is an honor to salute each member of the team.

John T. and Lillian G. Mathews, loyal friends of Mayo Clinic and founding benefactors of Heritage Hall, provided generous support that helped make this edition possible.

Special thanks to Dr. McConahey and his wife, Adrienne, to whom he dedicated the book. The warmth of their friendship remains a valued part of my experience working at Mayo Clinic. To their children—William McConahey, Peter McConahey and Meredith McConahey Pollak—my gratitude for endorsing this project and sharing their family artifacts. Peter McConahey was a longtime Mayo Clinic employee and member of the Heritage Days Committee. I admire Peter's dedication to Mayo's history and the insights he conveyed about his father's wartime experience.

I am grateful to Mark A. Warner, M.D., who wrote the Foreword, drawing upon his knowledge and advocacy for communicating medical and military history.

Thanks to colleagues in the Mayo Clinic Archive of the W. Bruce Fye Center for the History of Medicine and W. Bruce Fye History of Medicine Library for their expertise in researching and making available the rich historical resources of our institution: Christopher J. Boes, M.D., Emily C. Brown, Emily J. Christopherson, Karen F. Koka, Gioia R. Spatafora. Mona K. Stevermer, Alec J. Thicke, Brooke A. Weber, Ph.D., and Renee E. Ziemer.

This book is the latest example of a highly productive collaboration between Mayo Clinic Press and Mayo Clinic Heritage Days.

Mayo Clinic Press brings inspiring dedication and professionalism to our shared projects. My respect and admiration go to Daniel J. Harke, M.B.A., publisher; Nina E. Wiener, editor-in-chief; James R. Cahoy, principal product manager; Karen R. Wallevand, M.S., senior editor; Stewart (Jay) J. Koski, M.F.A., art director; Christine N. Boyer, associate product manager; and Kelly L. Hahn, marketing manager.

Thanks to Matthew C. Meyer for photographing artifacts from Dr. McConahey's military service. For the strongest visual impact, this volume includes black-and-white wartime photographs printed directly from historic negatives in the McConahey family collection.

It also captures the elegant design of the 1966 edition. James Eckman, Ph.D., of the Mayo Clinic editorial staff designed the typography for the Domesday Press, which he ran in the basement of his home during that pre-computer era.

Mayo Clinic Heritage Days championed the project as an exemplar of the Heritage Days mission to honor the history, culture and values of Mayo Clinic through creative efforts that engage contemporary audiences. The team delivered essential editorial and project management skills. Special thanks to Jeanne M. Klein, coordinator; Nicole L. Babcock, program specialist; and Trish M. Amundson, M.M., co-chair.

My wife, Lea C. Dacy, has been a constant support in this and every other endeavor I have undertaken at Mayo Clinic. Her encouragement is a blessing and her editorial judgment is a benefit that helps keep me out of trouble when it comes time to write.

To all, my heartfelt gratitude in making it possible to share, as Dr. Warner described, this "common-man storytelling, written by an uncommonly great man." Planning my own retirement now, I am keeping the handwritten note I received from Dr. McConahey, which he addressed to me as his friend.

MATTHEW D. DACY, M.A.
DIRECTOR, MAYO CLINIC HERITAGE HALL
AND CO-CHAIR, MAYO CLINIC HERITAGE DAYS

ABOUT THE AUTHOR

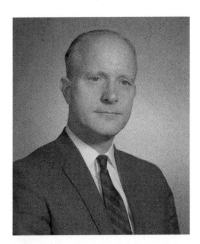

W ILLIAM M. MCCONAHEY, JR., WAS BORN ON May 7, 1916, in Pittsburgh, Pennsylvania. He received the B.A. degree in 1938 from Washington and Jefferson College and the M.D. degree in 1942 from Harvard University. He was an intern at Philadelphia General Hospital from 1942 to 1943.

During World War II, Dr. McConahey entered active duty on July 17, 1943, and served as a battalion surgeon in the Medical Corps of the U.S. Army, which is the subject of this book. Assigned to the 90th Infantry Division, he landed in the Allied assault against Nazi-held Europe on June 8, 1944, D-Day+2. Dr. McConahey served in France, Germany and Czechoslovakia and attained the rank of captain. *Battalion Surgeon* concludes with his honorable discharge on September 28, 1945.

Dr. McConahey began advanced medical training at Mayo Graduate School of Medicine (today, Mayo Clinic College of Medicine and Science) in 1946 and received the M.S. degree in medicine from the University of Minnesota in 1948. He was appointed a Mayo Clinic consultant in medicine in 1949 and served as chair of the Division of Endocrinology from 1968 to 1974. Dr. McConahey advanced through the academic ranks to become professor of medicine.

He had a special interest in diseases of metabolism and the endocrine system and published extensively in medical journals and textbooks. He received the Distinguished Service Award from the American Thyroid Association in 1973 and the Alumni Association of Washington and Jefferson College in 1978. Dr. McConahey retired from Mayo Clinic in December 1985 and died on April 22, 2004.